NECK DISSECTION – CLINICAL APPLICATION AND RECENT ADVANCES

Edited by **Raja Kummoona**

Neck Dissection – Clinical Application and Recent Advances
Edited by Raja Kummoona

Published by InTech
Janeza Trdine 9, 51000 Rijeka, Croatia

Publishing Process Manager Silvia Vlase

Technical Editor Teodora Smiljanic

Cover Designer InTech Design Team

Additional hard copies can be obtained from orders@intechopen.com

Neck Dissection – Clinical Application and Recent Advances,
Edited by Raja Kummoona
p. cm.
ISBN 978-953-51-0104-8

For EU product safety concerns:
IN TECH d.o.o., Prolaz Marije Krucifikse Kozulić 3, 51000 Rijeka, Croatia,
info@intechopen.com or visit our website at intechopen.com.

Meet the editor

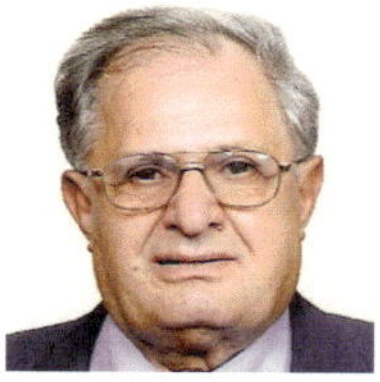

Professor Raja Kummoona, Fellow of the Royal College of Surgeons of England (FDSRCS), Emiratus professor of Maxillofacial Surgery of Iraqi Board for Medical Specializations, is one of 40 top scientist in Iraq. He has been a member of the Research Fellow Royal college of Surgeons of England (1975-1977), the President of Iraqi Dental Society (1977-1985). Prof. Kummoona has contributed to the field with a number of publications and also by advocating many surgical procedures. He has conducted research in cancer surgery, flap reconstruction, TMJ surgery and facial injuries caused by missiles.

Contents

Preface

Advances in the management of cervical lymph node deposit required many modalities in surgery, deep X-ray therapy and chemotherapy. In order to achieve maximal effectiveness when treating a patient, it is essential to take considerable criteria factors such as: the pathology of a particular tumor (beside the status of patient's general condition) and the anatomy of the region. It is important that the pathology is assessed by the surgeon and not by the pathologist.

The chosen title of the book is based on different techniques used for lymphadenactomy: radical neck dissection, selective neck dissection and conservative neck dissection, including the preservation of the spinal accessory nerve, internal jugular vein and sterno mastoid muscle, using techniques such as the endoscopic technique with reboot surgery and other types of incisions. Recently the design of the lateral cervical flap proved to be an excellent access for different modalities of lymph adenactomy.

The treatment of the majority of patients with lymph node metastasis required a multidisciplinary approach. The joined efforts of the surgeon, radiotherapist, oncologist and pathologist are necessary for a successful outcome. They should all be involved in the treatment plan and should understand the principle and current applications of chemotherapy and radiotherapy in neck cancer metastasis.

The book comprises 11 chapters (including the Introductory chapter), which fall naturally into three main sections: I) History of neck dissection, II) Different techniques of neck dissection and Complications, III) Advances and modification of neck dissection.

This type of publication required a great support and effort both from the book editor and from the publishing team. I would like to extend my thanks and gratitude to Ms Natalia Reinic, editor relations consultant, and to the publishing process managers Ms Alenka Urbancic, Mr Marko Rebrovic and Ms Silvia Vlase. All these people spent a lot of time into making this book a worthwhile publication and interesting to the readers and top specialist concerned with neck dissection.

Prof. Raja Kummoona
Professor Emeritus of Maxillofacial Surgery
Acting Chairman of Maxillofacial Surgery
Iraqi Board for Medical Specializations
Baghdad, Iraq

Head and Neck Cancer and Neck Dissection - A Personal View

Raja Kummoona
Professor Emeritus of Maxillofacial Surgery,
Acting Chairman of Maxillofacial Surgery,
Iraqi Board for Medical Specializations,
Baghdad,
Iraq

Head and neck cancer represent nearly 12% of total malignancies, including the face, the oropharynx, the parotid gland and other salivary glands, the orbit, the jaw , the sinuses and other parts of the face including the skin. These anatomical sites might be affected by other varieties of cancer, such as basal cell carcinoma, squamous-cell carcinoma, fibro sarcoma, osteogenic sarcoma and jaw lymphoma, and non-Hodgkin's lymphoma and Hodgkin's lymphoma. Jaw lymphoma is nominated from other parts of the world and Africa, such as Burkitt lymphoma. Jaw lymphoma is quite different from Burkitt lymphoma in its clinical features, aetiology and even with regard to its treatment. Jaw lymphoma is presented as having a very rapid onset with a fast spread to internal organs and the brain, while Burkitt lymphoma is a slowly growing tumour; it is well known that Burkitt lymphoma can be treated successfully by a few courses of cyclophosphamide (40 mg/square meter) but jaw lymphoma requires a more complicated regimen with combination of many chemotherapeutic agents, such as CHOP(therapeutic regimen of jaw lymphoma consist of eight doses over 24 weeks including 1.5mg/m^2 Vincristine,50mg/m^2 Adriamycin, 1000mg/m^2 Cyclophosphomide, 10mg/m^2 Methotroxate and 50mg/m^2 prednisolone) and it rarely deposits its tumour to the lymph nodes. Cancer of the head and neck constitute an important section of the total cancers affecting the body, and oral cancer represents about 4% of this; it is not necessary that all such cancers have nodal deposits in the neck, such jaw lymphoma or Burkitt Lymphoma. Malignant tumours such as squamous cell carcinoma - which form about 95% of oral cancers - and Melanoma - a highly malignant tumour with early metastasis - are rare and aggressive types of tumours and the survival rate is very low. Other malignant tumours, such as adenocarcinoma - which is a slowly growing malignant tumour - have less of a tendency for cervical node metastasis.

Cancer of the paranasal sinuses is considered to be an aggressive type of malignancy with a tendency to invade the orbit and the base of the skull. The most common tumour of the sinuses is squamous cell carcinoma rather than adenocarcinoma, as a result of cellular changes from respiratory columnar type to squamous type due to the recurrence of infection and other irritating agents. These types of tumour metastasise in the cervical lymph nodes. Cancer of the oral cavity represents somewhat less than 4% of total cancer incidence but this might increase to more than 40% - as in India due to dietary causes such as spicy foods and smoking - and these tumours appear as a fissure or exophytic growth or ulcer with white leukoplakia, and the most common site which is affected is the tongue and floor of the mouth. Both of these lesions in early metastasis affect the deep chain of the cervical lymph nodes, and the managements of these cases was based on a combination of three modalities in the form of radical surgery, chemotherapy and deep x-ray therapy. There is no possibility of a single technique for treatment in these cases. A frozen section in theatre is required for any assessment of the complete eradication of tumours

Nowadays, chemotherapy has played an important role in the management of head and neck cancers due to advances in the manufacturing of these drugs and DXT (deep x-ray therapy) which have become more specific and more precise in targeting cancer tumours. One technique of note is the use of the gamma Knife (Cobalt 60) in the management of brain tumours and intraocular malignancies without evisceration of the eye ball (which can be very depressing and inconvenient for patients).

The advancement of surgical management of head and neck tumours was based on advances in flap surgeries, such as a pedicle flaps like the forehead flap, the lateral cervical flap, the deltopectoral flap and the trapezius flap, or else by using free flaps like the forearm flap and the tapes dorsalis flap; these flaps are required for microanastomosis for the reconstruction the surgical defects after radical cancer surgery. We have not forgotten that the traditional use of radical neck dissection as a method of treatment for cervical lymph node metastasis has not often been used as a surgical procedure for the total radical excision of cervical lymph nodes with the radical excision of the sternomastoid muscle, the accessory nerve, deep cervical fascia and internal jugular vein ligation. This procedure has become less popular due to the creation of an obvious vertical band of scars extending all over the neck and dropping off the shoulder with a superficial exposure of the carotid tree just below the skin. This problem was overcome by the advancement of the trapezius flap so as to cover the carotid tree and so avoid any traumatic injuries to carotid content. These complications have been avoided by advances in other techniques, such as selective neck dissection, functional neck dissection and supraomohyoid neck dissection.

The advancements of different diagnostic tools for detection of any cervical lymph node metastasis and assessment of these deposit been used by application of ultra sonography , MRI and CT scan with protocol for management of cervical lymph nodes metastasis is the basis for management of cervical lymph node metastasis.

The most common malignant tumours of the orofacial region is basal cell carcinoma affecting the skin of the face and this is more common among white people who have less melanin pigment in their skin and who have continuous exposure to sun light. This tumour is a slowly growing type with a tendency to invade the underlying structures and it does not metastasis to the cervical lymph nodes. Squamous cell carcinoma represents about 95% of the total oral malignancies mainly affecting the tongue and the floor of the mouth with tendency for cervical lymph node deposits. The management of these tumours requires the application of all modalities of treatment, surgery, DXT and chemotherapy.

Adenocarcinoma is less common in the oral cavity and affects the minor salivary glands - it is more common in the maxilla and it is a slowly growing tumour that rarely metastasises in the cervical lymph nodes and is less aggressive than adenocarcinoma of the gastro-intestinal tract, which is a highly malignant tumour with early metastasis in mesenteric lymph nodes. The eradication of these tumours is rather difficult due to their early metastasis and the complicated anatomy of the area, which makes radical surgery rather difficult. Recent advances in chemotherapy have seen the application of Gemzar (gencitabin) (this drug interferes with the growth and spread of cancer cells by inducing apoptosis and ant metabolite and also been used with Carboplatin) - which is a specific chemotherapy for this type of malignancy and was a promising type of chemotherapy even in cases of fourth-stage of pancreatic adenocarcinoma. In the parotid glands, adenocarcinoma is common and also is mucoepidermoid carcinoma and other malignancies; only rarely is the parotid affected by malignant oncocytoma, this type of tumour metastasises in cervical lymph nodes and requires radical resection of the tumour with chemotherapy and DXT.

The majority of head and neck tumours require neck dissection at once, affecting the oral cavity and parotid region. However, tumours affecting the middle third of the face - such as the maxilla or the orbit - require radical surgery with flap reconstruction followed by DXT and chemotherapy, rather than radical neck dissection and as there is rarely any metastasis in the cervical lymph nodes.

Melanoma of the orofacial tumour is a highly malignant type of tumour with a high tendency for early cervical metastasis, and the prognosis is not very promising. It requires multiple therapies for controlling its tumours, including chemotherapy and radical surgery, while melanoma of the lower limbs is less aggressive and responds to radical surgery and is diagnosed with lymphoscintigraphy.

Current cancer research focused now a days on understanding on the response and resistance to treatment and apoptosis. Cancer treatment depend not only on cellular damages as achieved by chemotherapy and DXT but also on the ability of the cell to respond to damages by inducing apoptotic changes and mutation in apoptotic pathway to end with resistance to chemotherapy drugs and radiation. Mitochondria and cell surface receptors

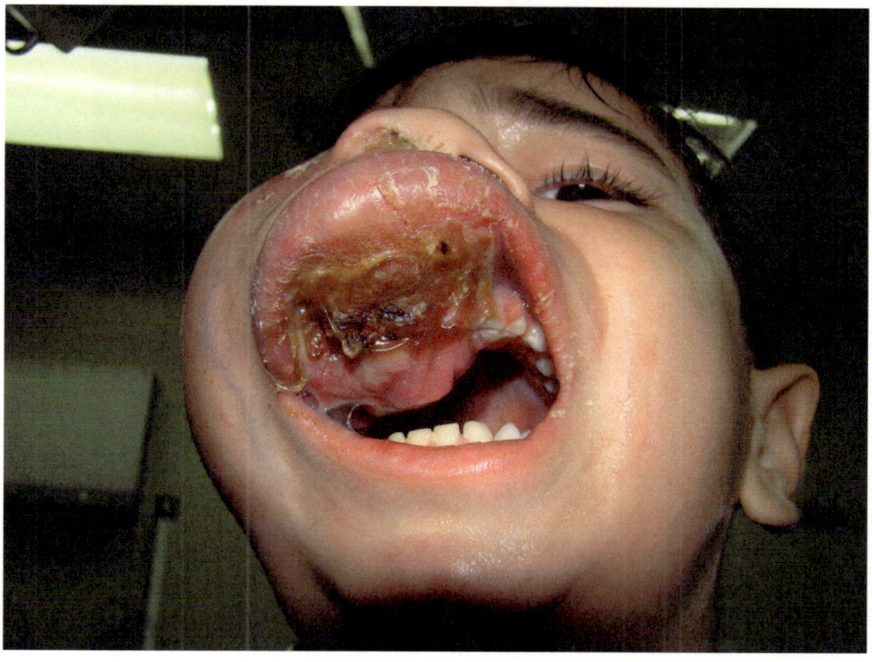

Fig. 1. Jaw lymphoma of the right side of the face of a 2 year old boy with a history of one month.

mediate the pathway of apoptosis and this pathways mediated by Bcl-2 family protein and the final excursion of cell death is performed by caspace cascade which is triggered by release cytochrome C from mitochondria. Most of the activity in the development of apoptosis drugs was concentrated on apoptosis inducers for treatment of malignancies.

The future might be very promising for the control of lymph node deposits by using different methods of accessing neck dissection as well as the recent application of robot surgery (the da Vinci surgical robot system) which is more widely used in prostatic eradication than in any other specialty and which might be used in general surgery. However, this technique is limited in its application in all fields and even in head and neck malignancies. Expanding the role of DXT and chemotherapy as the first line of treatment and as a curative therapy without the need for radical neck dissection, either as an adjuvant with surgery or without as in jaw lymphoma (which is the only line of treatment for such a highly malignant tumour, being a fast spreading and fatal tumour).

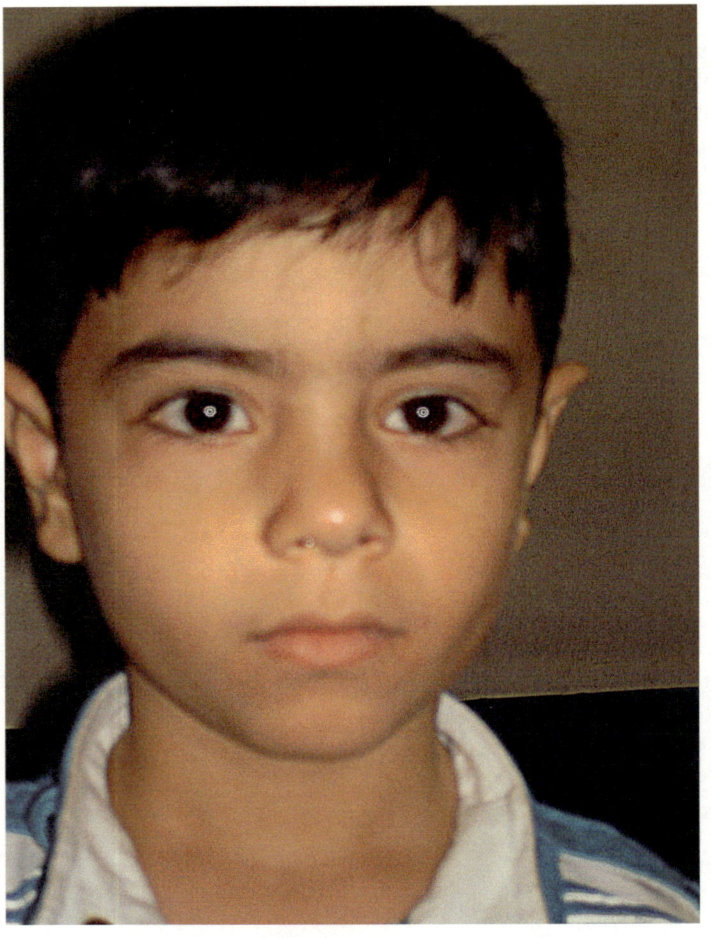

Fig. 2. Post-therapy after 2 years of treatment of jaw lymphoma by 6 courses of chemotherapy, with the collaboration with Prof. Selma Al Hadad, Paediatric Oncologist, Medical City Baghdad.

Part 1

History of Neck Dissection

1

A Brief History of Cervical Lymphadenectomy

Jeremiah C. Tracy
Tufts Medical Center,
Department of Otolaryngology – Head and Neck Surgery
USA

1. Introduction

Head and neck cancer is an aggressive disease with substantial morbidity associated with local invasion and regional lymphatic spread. Local spread through lymphatic channels is the most common course of disease progression; and nodal disease is often regarded as the most important prognostic factor in malignancy of the head and neck. [Ferlito 2006, Shah] It has been estimated that the presence of lymphatic metastases indicates a 50% decrease in survival; with contralateral nodal disease indicating another 50% decrease. [Leemans 1993, 1994]

Neck dissection describes a procedure involving the en bloc removal of some or all of the lymphatic organs of the head and neck. In current practice the procedure is often performed simultaneously with resection of a primary tumor of the head and neck. The scope of the resection is quite variable and, throughout history, has been a source of some debate. In 1988 the American Head and Neck Society formed a task group to synthesize a standard nomenclature regarding neck dissection, their recommendations have gained near universal acceptance throughout North America and internationally as well. [Robbins 1991, 2002, 2008]

Currently the American Head and Neck Society classifies cervical lympadenectomy into 4 categories:

1. Radical neck dissection
2. Modified radical neck dissection
3. Selective neck dissection
4. Extended neck dissection

A radical neck dissection is defined as en bloc excision of lymph node levels I-V (Figure 1) along with the internal jugular vein (IJV), sternocleidomastoid muscle (SCM), and spinal accessory nerve (SAN). A modified radical neck dissection also involves the complete removal of levels I-V but with sparing of one or more of the nonlymphatic structures (IJV, SCM, SAN). A selective neck dissection is defined as a procedure that removes anything other than levels I-V. The nomenclature of selective neck dissection assumes that IJV, SCM, and SAN are all preserved unless otherwise noted. The specific levels removed are listed in parentheses (ie. SND [I-III]). Finally, an extended neck dissection is any procedure that removes additional structures beyond those involved in a radical neck dissection, for example superior mediastinal lymph nodes, or the external carotid artery. Very complete and specific recommendations regarding classification and terminology are clearly laid out in publications by Robbins et al. [Robbins 1991, 2002, 2008]

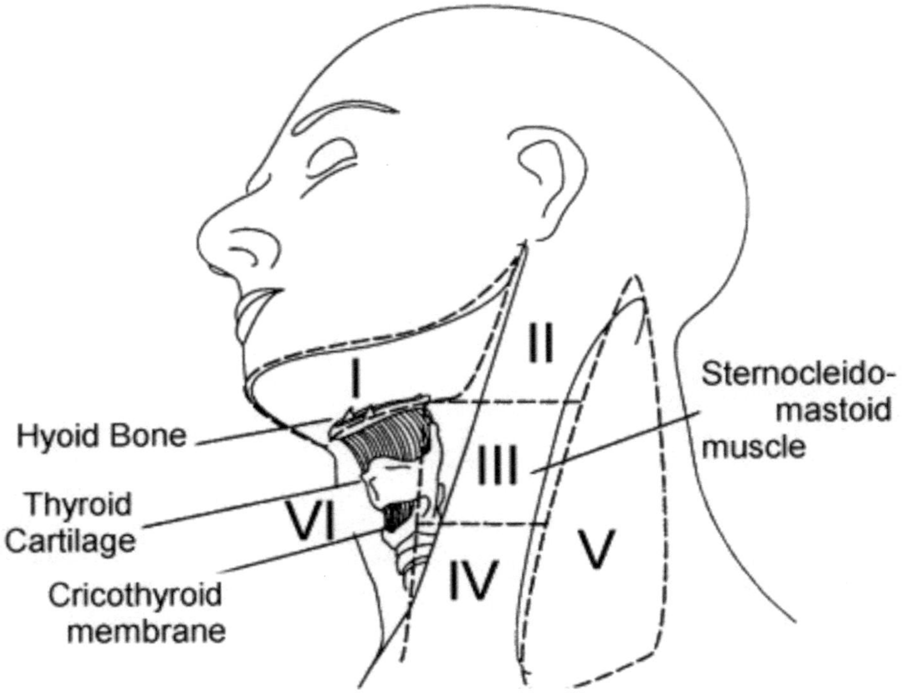

Fig. 1. Lymph node levels of the neck, as first defined and applied by the Memorial Hospital head and neck service. [website]

There is still no strict consensus regarding the indications for each type of procedure, however some broad guidelines do exist. Generally speaking, radical neck dissection is recommended in the management of recurrent disease or disease that grossly involves associated non-lymphatic structures. Modified radical neck dissection has become the standard treatment of clinically apparent neck disease. Selective neck dissection is generally used when elective neck dissection is performed, that is, treatment of patients with no clinical evidence of neck disease but a primary tumor that is high risk for lymphatic spread. Recent studies have supported the application of selective neck dissection in treating clinically apparent disease as well. [Robbins 2004, 2005]

Squamous cell carcinoma accounts for more than 85% of malignancy of the upper aerodigestive tract. Neck dissection is most frequently performed as a treatment for squamous cell carcinoma, however it is also utilized in most other types of head and neck malignancy. Aside from squamous cell carcinoma, neck dissection is often employed in the management of thyroid, cutaneous, and salivary malignancy.

2. Early history

The importance of cervical lymphatic disease has been recognized for well over one hundred years. Indeed, many surgeons of the 19th century regarded neck disease in mucosal cancers as an indication of incurability. Surgical treatment of malignant tumors of the neck have been described as far back as the early 1800's, generally with significant patient mortality associated. [Rinaldo 2008, Folz 2007, 2008]. Maximilian von Chelius famously stated "once the growth in the mouth has spread to the submaxilary gland, complete removal of the disease is impossible." [Chelius 1847] In order to treat lymphatic metastases, physicians and scientists had first to realize a modern paradigm of medicine.

Prior to the 18th century, western medicine was dominated by the humoral theory of disease. A lack of understanding of the nature of malignant disease and its spread through lymphatic channels would certainly make the principles of modern neck dissection elusive. Humoralism is a theory of medicine often attributed to Hippocrates, although it probably had its roots in older civilizations of Egypt or Assyria. The basis of humoralism is that there are four essential humors of the human body: blood, phlegm, black bile, and yellow bile. Disease is the imbalance of these humors and treatments aimed at restoring balance by medication or by letting of one or more of the humors.[Sudhoff] This philosophy was embraced by Galen and other scientists of western medicine until the 15th and 16th centuries. (Figure 2) During this time dissections and experiments by Andreus Vesalius, William

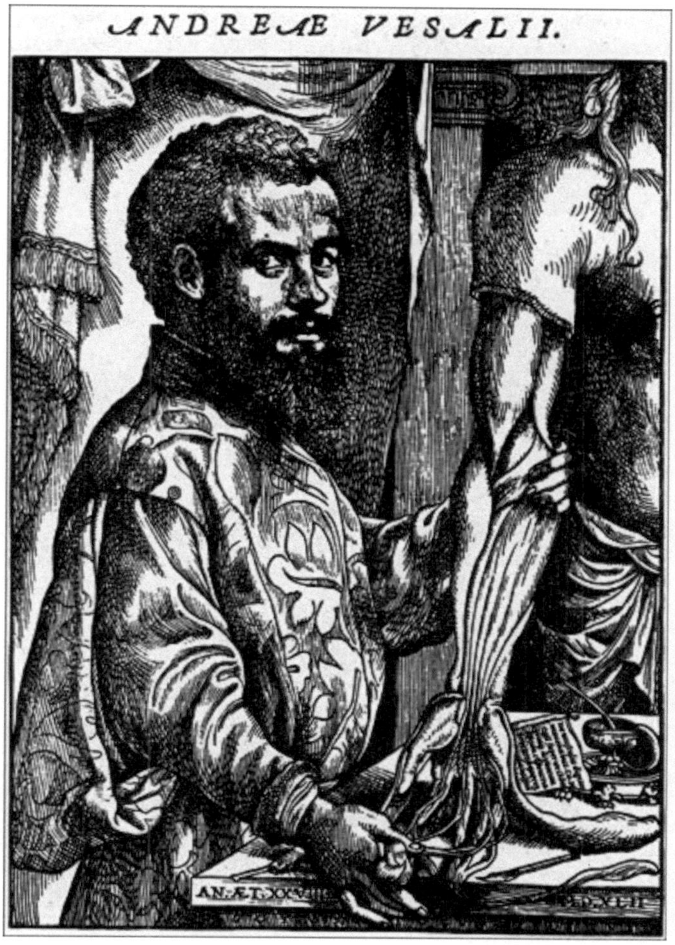

Fig. 2. Portrait of Andreas Vesalius; reproduced from *De Humani Corporis Fabrica,* Volume 1. Vesalius' contributions in the field of anatomy led Renaissance scientists to reconsider many fundamental principles of the earlier Hippocratic medicine. [Vesalius]

Harvey, and other greats of the scientific revolution began to shed doubt on many of the essential principles of Hippocratic medicine. [Folz 2008, Harvey, Shapin] Advances in science and technology ultimately led to Virchow's proposal of "cell theory" at the turn of the 19th century. [Virchow] Modern biology has been built upon the principles of cell theory. The mid 19th century also saw two great leaps forward in the progress of surgery. In 1846 John Collins Warren performed a neck mass excision at Massachusetts General Hospital under general anesthesia using ether (Figure 3). This well-publicized event marks the birth of modern general anesthesia, which has allowed longer more extensive surgeries, more delicate dissection and hemodynamic control; not to mention the benefit to patient comfort. [Folz 2007, Major] The second well-documented surgical development of the era was Joseph Lister's proposal that infection is caused by spread of microorganisms. He demonstrated that by maintaining sterile technique using antiseptics like phenol and carbolic acid; one could drastically reduce the rate of surgical site infections. [Lister]

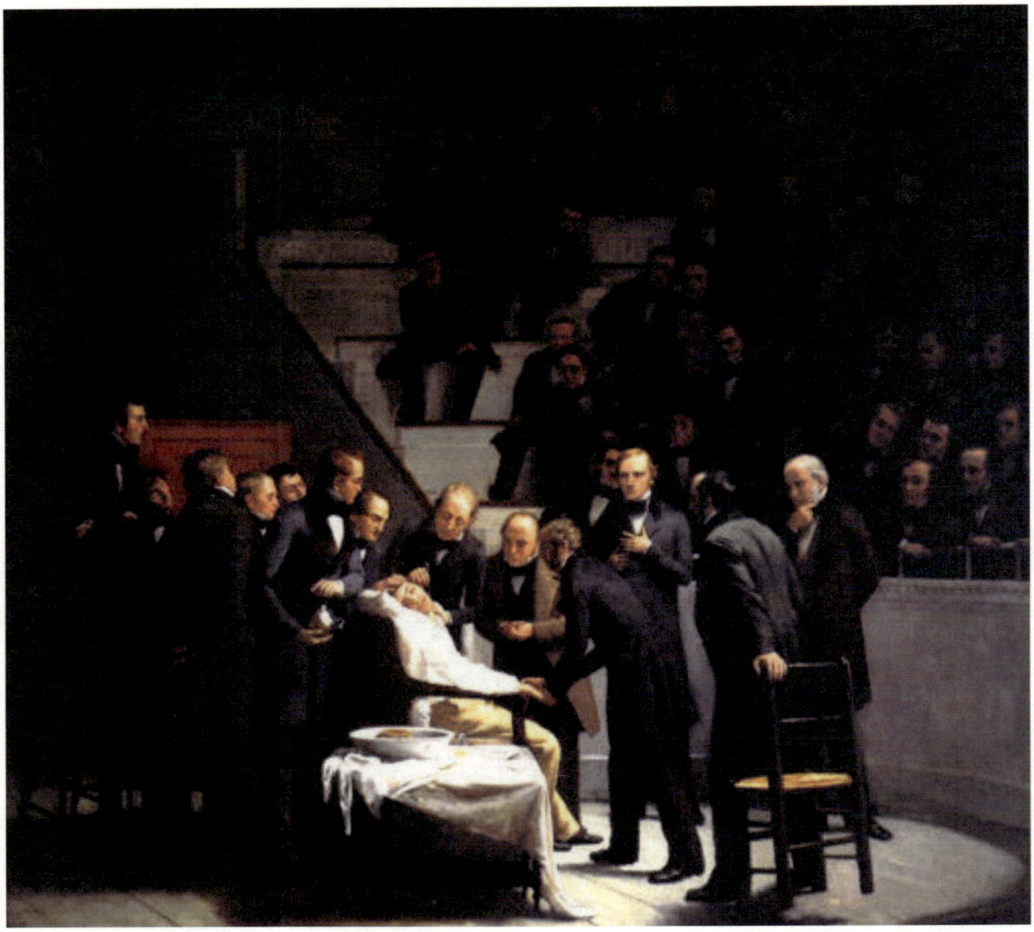

Fig. 3. John Collins Warren performs the first neck surgery on a patient under general anesthesia at Massachusetts General Hospital 1846. "The First Operation Under Ether" oil painting by John Cutler Hinckley.

The 1800's also, and not coincidentally, mark the same era in which head and neck oncology was first accurately recognized and described. That is, the recognition that neck disease represents lymphatic spread from primary malignancy of the upper aerodigestive tract. It was in the late 1800's that the first modern descriptions of neck dissection are documented. When and who performed the first neck dissection is a subject of some controversy [Ferlito 2007, Towpik 1990] Rinaldo recently documented the early history of neck dissection well in a paper that highlighted early attempts at en bloc cervical lymphadenectomy by what he termed "the four giants of 19th century surgery" (Kocher, Billroth, von Langenbeck, and von Volkmann). These publications generally described removal of malignant neck masses, with or without an associated primary tumor. They represent single cases or small case serious, and they generally describe tumor excision rather than a planned resection of cervical lymphatics. In this era of neck dissection, outcomes were quite poor. [Rinaldo 2007, Kocher 1880, Langenbeck 1875]

One candidate for first neck dissection was described in an 1880 publication by Emil Theodor Kocher. [Kocher] Kocher described his now well-known "y-shaped" incision in order to remove upper neck lymphatics en bloc with the submandibular gland and oral cavity primary tumors. Kocher advocated for the systematic removal of the submandibular gland and associated lymph nodes in addition to the primary site when performing floor of mouth and tongue resections through a transcervical approach. This is distinct from earlier publications by Warren and von Langenbeck that were aimed at simply removing a discrete neck tumor. [Warren 1837, Langenbeck 1875]

The eponym "Kocher incision" (Figure 4) to describe this approach to oral cancer was first coined by Henry T. Butlin, who has been called "the father of British head and neck surgery." [Uttley 2000] In a landmark publication, Butlin presented a case series on the surgical management of tongue cancer. [Butlin 1885] In this paper he demonstrated that patients who underwent resection of submandibular lymph nodes (regardless of lymphatic spread at the time of operation) had better recurrence and survival outcomes than those that

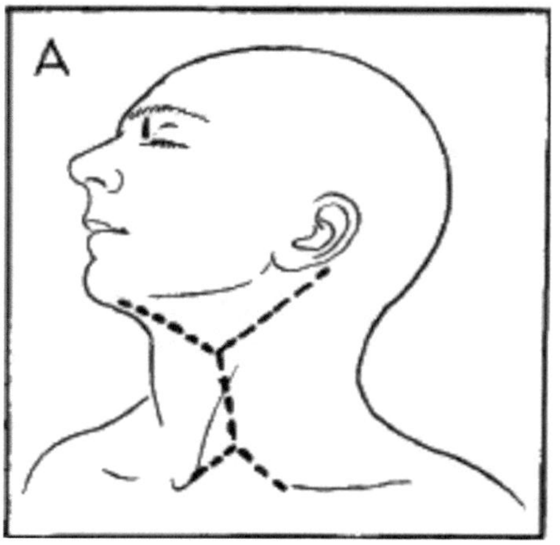

Fig. 4. The Kocher incision describes a y-shaped incision with the long arm running along the anterior border of the SCM, extending from the mastoid tip to the clavicle; and the short arm extending anteriorly to allow full exposure of the submandibular triangle. Above, the Martin modification maintains obtuse-angled skin flaps for better perfusion at the flap tips, also a second inferior "y" to allow greater supraclavicular exposure.

did not. In the paper he strongly advocated for "prophylactic" (what today would be described as elective) resection of submandibular lymph nodes in all cases of tongue cancer. This likely was the start of one of the great questions that still persists in modern head and neck oncology: when to treat the clinically negative neck.

Most recent publications recognize Jawdynski of Poland as the first to perform a radical neck dissection. In 1888 he published the report of cervical lymphadenectomy involving all lymphatics from the mandible to the sternum as well as the internal jugular vein, sternocleidomastoid, and spinal accessory nerve. This case also involved ligation of the common carotid artery as the tumor was invading this structure. The procedure described is indeed quite similar if not identical to a current radical neck dissection. Unfortunatly Jawdynski published few other works. His career was cut short when he died of infection at the young age of 45. [Towpik 1990]

3. The early 20th century

At the beginning of the 20th century George Crile of the United States published a series of cases of "cervical lymphadenectomy," performed to manage lymphatic spread of head and neck malignancies. The data was first presented in the 1905 annual Transactions of the Southern Surgical and Gynecologic Society. Later, it received national (and international) attention after being published in the Journal of the American Medical Association in 1906. [Crile 1905,1906] The paper reported a series of 132 cases. It included illustrations and a detailed description of the procedure (Figure 5). Subsequently the eponym "Crile procedure" was attached to cervical lymphadenectomy in the United States for several decades. The paper demonstrates a thorough understanding of cervical lymphatic spread, with the basic surgical principles based largely on Halsted's work in the field of breast surgery.

Crile's paper included a thoughtful discussion of the management of head and neck lymphatic disease, advocating for en bloc excision of all superficial lymphatic's of the neck in cases of clinical disease. Although credited with inventing the radical neck dissection, Crile proposed more limited lymphadenectomy in cases of clinically negative lymph nodes, or when non-lymphatic structures were not clearly involved in the surgical specimen. The data presented supports improved outcomes in terms of both recurrence and survival in patients who underwent radical neck dissection vs selective neck dissection (of course modern terminology was not used). In the subgroup with clinically positve neck disease and at least 3-year follow up, Crile observed an 18% (9/48) vs 75% (9/12) survival rate in those that underwent selective versus radical neck dissection. [Crile 1906]

Aside from the controversy regarding whether or not Crile is truly to be credited with performing the first neck dissection, the importance of this paper is agreed a upon. At the time of its publication, Crile's was the largest series available on the subject of neck dissection. Further, Crile included a discussion of the question of elective neck dissection. Crile was generally in favor of elective treatment, citing the previous work of Butlin (although Crile's data did not address the issue directly). Most importantly, Crile's paper included an analysis that indicated improved outcomes when neck dissection was performed as a complete en bloc cervical lymphadenectomy, rather than removing only grossly diseased nodes. Simply put, Crile recognized that treatment of malignant neck disease must involve complete cervical lymphadenectomy rather than simply excising those cervical lymph nodes that were grossly diseased. He further provided data in a relatively large case series supporting this claim. In this way Crile proposed the first standardized treatment algorithm in the management of lymphatic metastases of the head and neck.

Based largely on Crile's observations, the 20th century was characterized by a movement towards more aggressive management of clinical lymphatic desease. Blair and Brown demonstrated an increasingly intricate understanding of the disease process and discussed a large series of cases. Their paper was the first to report a standardized application of radiation therapy in treating cervical nodal disease, although the role of radiation at that time was exclusively one of salvage therapy. Their 1933 publication gave quite detailed descriptions of the surgical techniques, as well as indications and contraindications (Figure 6). The authors also outlined criteria for "unresectability" that were surprisingly similar to those employed today.

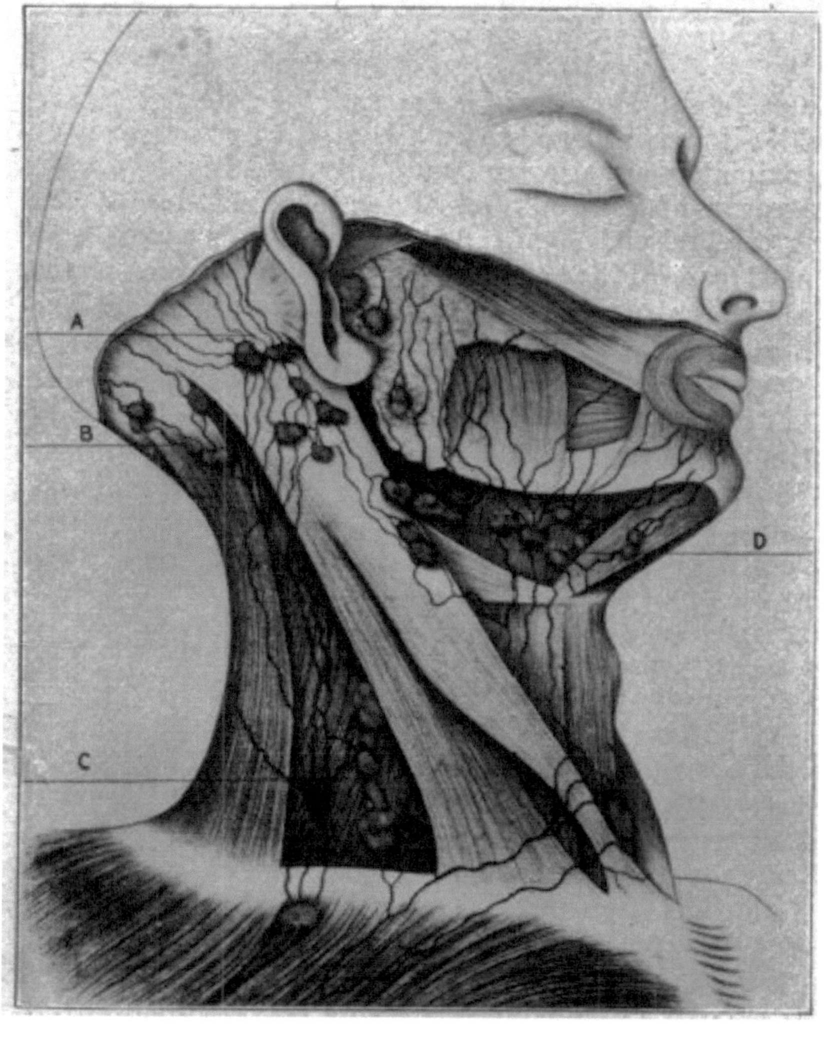

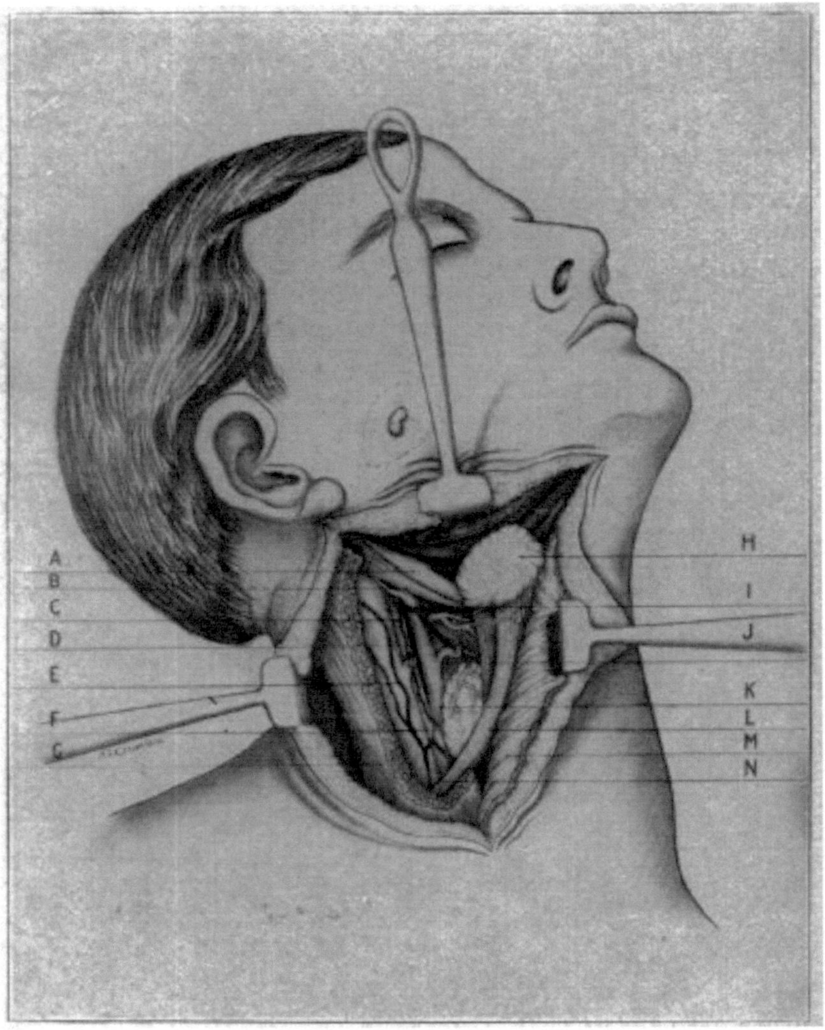

Fig. 5. A. Superficial lymph nodes of the neck by George Crile. B. Diagram of a neck dissection performed on a patient with a cutaneous malignancy.

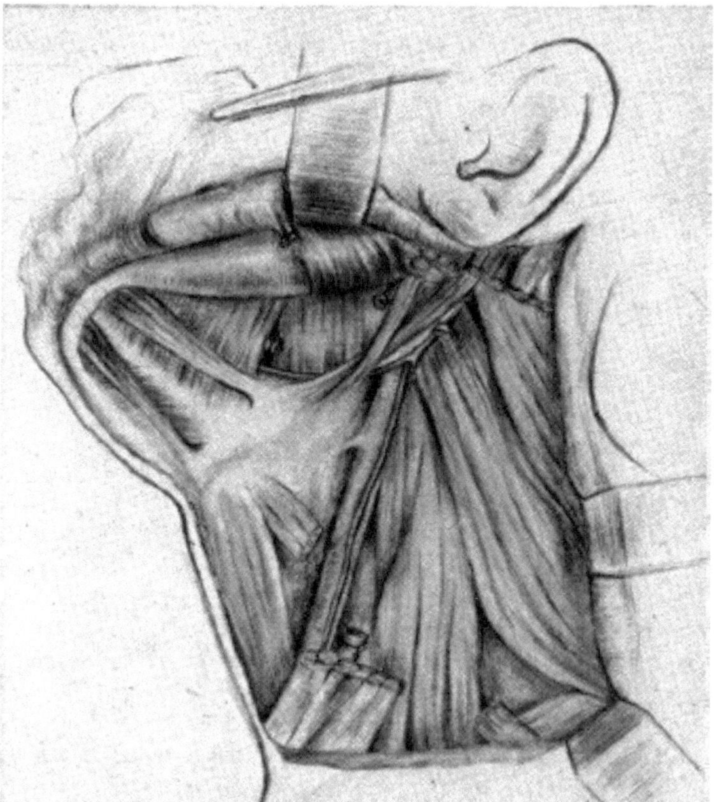

Fig. 6. Surgical field after neck dissection from Blair and Brown. Note a radical neck dissection with removal of SAN, SCM, IJV, and submandibular gland has been performed.

4. Controversy regarding technique and application

In 1951 Hayes Martin published his landmark paper, reporting on 1450 Cases performed at Memorial Hospital in New York over a 22 year period. Martin argued unequivocally for radical neck dissection in all cases of nodal disease: "In our opinion the partial operation should never be used." Regarding preservation of the spinal accessory nerve: "After repeated observations of the surgical anatomy of this nerve in relation to the upper portion of the internal jugular chain of lymphatic's, we are unalterably opposed to any attempt to preserve the nerve itself." The paper did not address recurrence rates between radical versus modified or selective neck dissections as it was practice at Memorial Hospital to perform radical neck dissection on all patients with clinical neck disease (Figure 7). The data presented demonstrated a much lower peri-operative mortality rate than previous publications: 1-2%. However it supported the previously documented high mortality associated with head and neck cancer in general, citing that 50% of the 334 patients who underwent isolated neck dissection were dead of disease at 5 years. [Martin 1951]

Martin's paper included publication of data from a survey that was sent to head and neck surgeons regarding opinions on the indications for elective neck dissection. Ultimately the data reflected extreme variation between surgeons. Martin concluded that his data generally support a role for elective surgery for primary tongue cancer, with more dubious indications in cases of laryngeal disease. Ultimately, however, this publication left the role of elective neck dissection unsettled.

The question of staged versus simultaneous radical neck dissection was also addressed. Earlier authors (including Crile cited above) noted high risk of increased intracranial pressure in patients undergoing bilateral internal jugular vein ligation simultaneously. [Sugarbaker, Crile] Martin's series included 66 patients who underwent simultaneous bilateral neck dissection, none of whom suffered peri-operative mortality. The recommendation based on this series was that neck dissections be staged by 3 weeks if disease permits, however if excision of the primary site requires exposure of both sides of the neck then neck dissection was performed simultaneously.

The direct language used in Martin's paper regarding radical versus partial neck dissection reflected a great controversy in the field of head and neck surgery. There remained many head and neck surgeons who commonly performed more limited neck dissection. Suarez is generally regarded as developing the functional neck dissection, a technique of cervical lymphadenectomy very similar to what is currently described as modified radical or selective neck dissection. [Suarez 1963, Ferlito 2005, Bocca 1964] Suarez' publication in 1963 demonstrated comparable levels of regional disease control with significantly decreased morbidity after these more conservative procedures. Suarez' paper contributed a very sophisticated description of the lymphatic drainage of the head and neck (Figure 8). It accurately described the different drainage patterns typical of head and neck malignancy based on primary tumor location.

Suarez' paper may be pinpointed as the start of a movement that has occurred in the later half of the 20th century towards modified radical and selective neck dissections.

In 1978 Jesse, Ballantyne, et al compared radical neck dissection with neck dissection that spared the spinal accessory nerve. They found no discrepancy in rate of disease recurrence between these two groups, even when controlling for disease severity. [Jesse 1978] Later, various studies comparing radical to various degrees of modified radical neck dissection demonstrated comparable rates of recurrence. [Spiro JD 1998, Byers 1988] Refinements in the field of radiation oncology likely allowed for this experimentation, as the availability and efficacy of radiation salvage therapy allowed for more conservative surgical practices. [Mendenhall 1995]

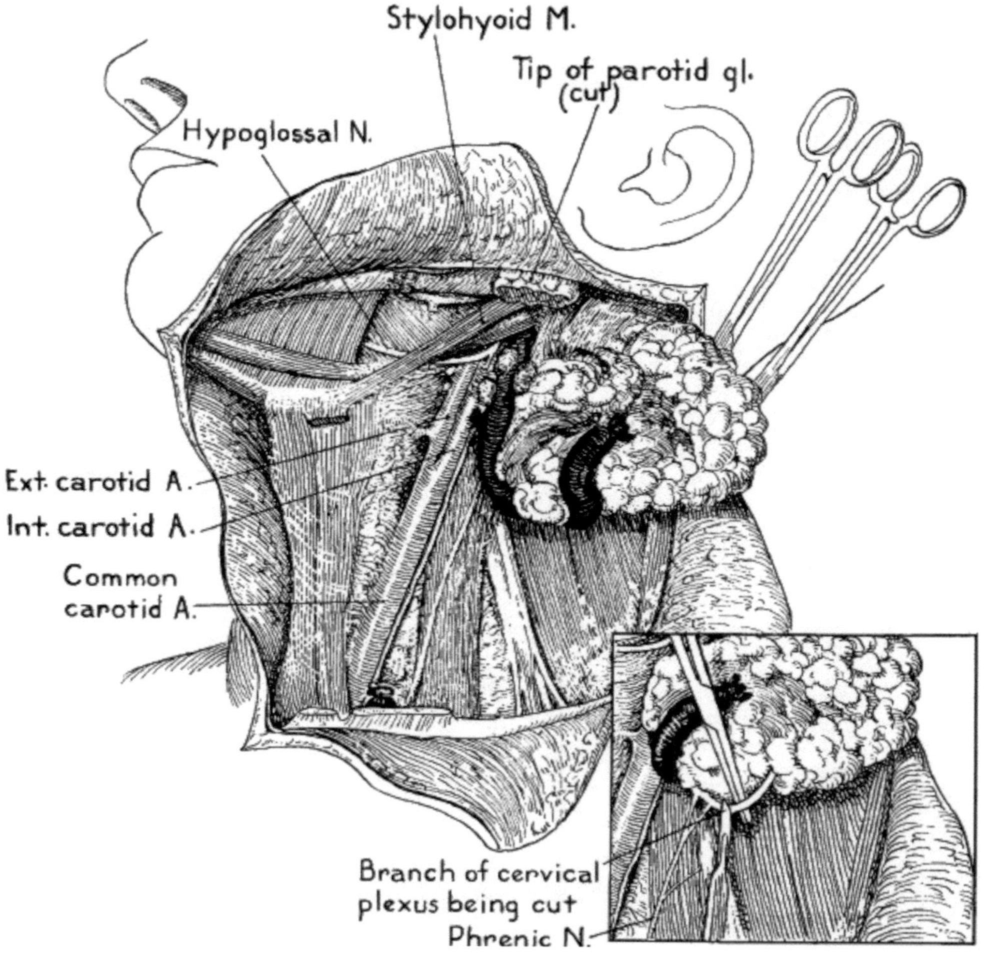

Fig. 7. En bloc removal of radical neck dissection specimen from Martin et al 1951. [Martin 1951]

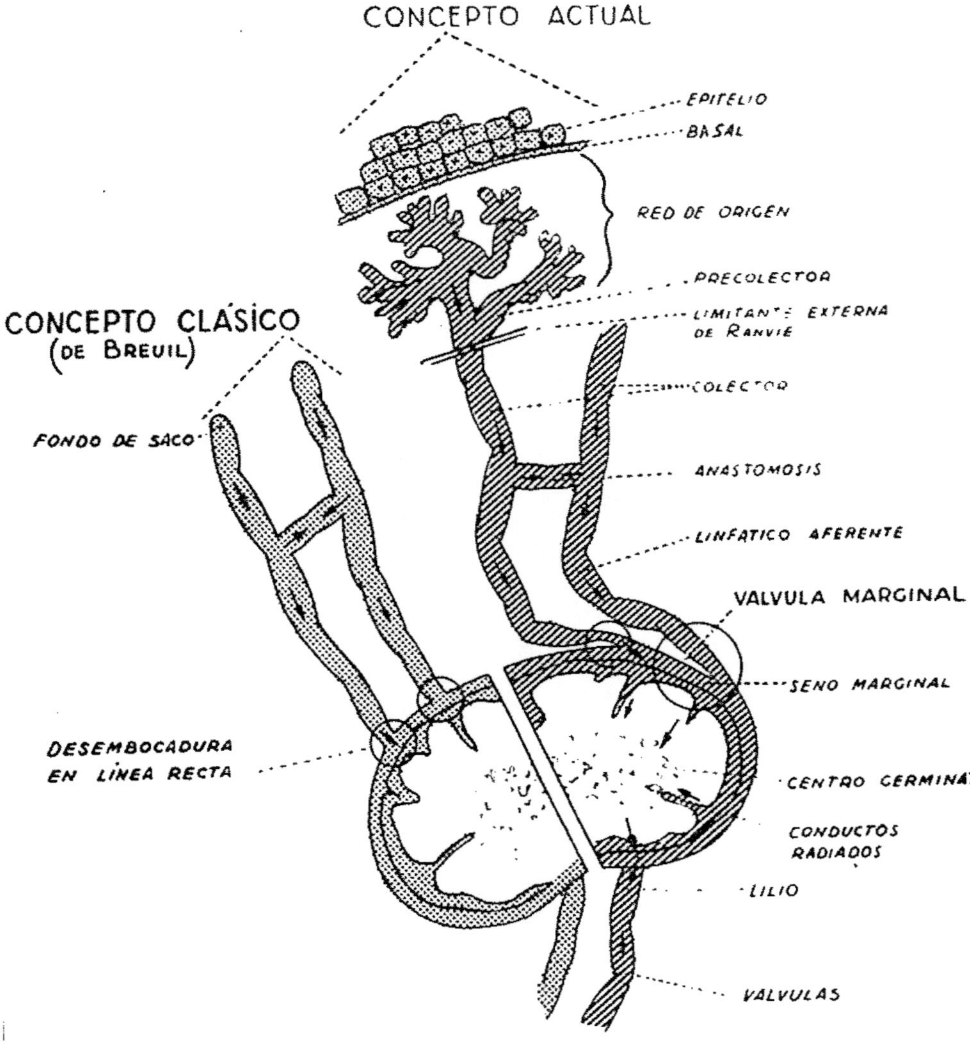

Fig. 8. A diagram of microscopic lymphatic anatomy from Suarez 1963. [Suarez 1963]

The basis of modern selective neck dissection lies in a sophisticated understanding of lymphatic drainage patterns of the head and neck. The contribution of Suarez was described above. In 1972 Robert M. Lindberg published a report on the surgical pathologic specimens from neck dissections. Lindberg reviewed 2,044 surgical specimens from the MD Anderson Cancer Institute in Texas; and reported the ditribution of pathologically positive nodes. This data set provided a wealth of knowledge regarding pattern of lymphatic spread based on primary site as well as tumor stage classification. His results supported many of Suarez' earlier recommendations and have led to our current guidelines regarding the application of selective neck dissection.

5. Current practice and future directions

In 1991 the American Head and Neck Society published guidelines regarding classification and nomenclature of neck dissection that have gained acceptance throughout much of the world. Under those guidelines all procedures are classified as radical neck dissection, modified radical neck dissection, selective neck dissection, and extended neck dissection (as described above). The current indications (and contraindications) to neck dissection are very much intertwined with the definitions of the procedures themselves.

There remains a great deal of variation regarding the application of these procedures in the management of head and neck cancer. Common areas of discrepancy include the role of elective neck dissection, modified radical versus therapeutic selective neck dissection, bilateral versus unilateral neck dissection and the timing in cases of bilateral surgery. A thorough description of the current nomenclature and indications for neck dissection are outside the scope of this chapter, however in reviewing the history of neck dissection; there is much to be learned regarding the current guidelines in cervical lymphadenectomy.

Spread to local lymph nodes is the course of disease progression in head and neck malignancy. Neck disease is a key prognostic factor with regards to recurrence after treatment as well as overall survival. Even with refined radiation therapy techniques available, the primary management of lymphatic disease is surgical resection. Procedures aimed at partial or complete cervical lymphadenectomy have been performed at least since the mid 19th century, with varying degrees of success. The current standard of care in head and neck oncology is a product of the history outlined above. In the case of neck dissection, we can see how the course of events shapes our understanding of a disease and our attempts at its eradication.

The current era is a very exciting time in head and neck oncology. Technology has grown at an exponential rate over recent decades and we, as clinicians, are still struggling to apply these resources to medical care. Much has been learned over the previous centuries but there are daunting obstacles yet to overcome. Important areas of current research include the expanding role of chemotherapy and radiation therapy in head and neck cancer. [Wolf 1990] Further, microbiologic techniques such as polymerase chain reaction and immunohistochemical staining have enabled researchers to identify microscopic foci of disease in surgical specimens. The way that this information should be applied to treatment has yet to be determined. Other procedures such as lymphoscintigraphy have become standard of care in other malignant diseases such as breast cancer and melanoma, however the utility in head an neck oncology has yet to be defined.

Neck dissection has been a vital aspect of head and neck cancer treatment since neoplastic disease was first described. Current studies in technology, radiation, and epidemiology will allow us to further perfect the technique and application of this procedure.

6. References

Blair VP, Brown JP. The treatment of cancerous or potentially cancerous cervical lymph nodes. Ann Surg 1933;98:650–61.

Bocca E. E´ videment "fonctionel" du cou dans la the´ rapie de principe des metastases ganglionnaires du cancer du larynx (Introduction a` la pre´ sentation d'un film). J Fr Oto-rhinolaryngol 1964;13:721–3.

Byers RM, Wolf PF, Ballantyne AJ. Rationale for elective modified neck dissection. Head Neck Surg 1988;10:160–7.

Crile GW. Excision of cancer of the head and neck. With special reference to the plan of dissection based on one hundred and thirtytwo operations. JAMA 1906;47:1780–6.

Crile GW. On the surgical treatment of cancer of the head and neck. With a summary of one hundred and twenty-one operations performed upon one hundred and five patients. Trans South Surg Gynecol Assoc 1905;18:108 - 27.

Chelius JM, South JF. A System of Surgery. Tr. from the German and accompanied with additional notes and observations by John F. South, vol. III. Philadelphia: Lea & Blanchard; 1847. p. 515.

Deschler DG and Day T. Pocket Guide to TNM Staging of Head and Neck Cancer and Neck Dissection Classification. Alexandria, VA. American Academy of Otolaryngology - Head and Neck Surgery; 2008.

Ferlito A, Rinaldo A. Neck dissection: historical and current concepts. Am J Otolaryngol. 2005;26:289–295.

Ferlito A, Rinaldo A, Silver CE, Shah JP, Suarez C, Medina JE, Kowalski LP, Johnson JT, Strome M, Rodrigo JP, Werner JA, Takes RP, Towpik E, Robbins KT, Leemans CR, Heranz J, Gavilan J, Shaha JR, Wei WI. Neck dissection: then and now. Auris Nasus Larynx. 2006; Vol 33: 365-374.

Ferlito A, Johnson JT, Rinaldo A, Pratt LW, Fagan JJ, Weir N, Suárez C, Folz BJ, Bień S, Towpik E, Leemans CR, Bradley PJ, Kowalski LP, Herranz J, Gavilán J, Olofsson J.

European surgeons were the first to perform neck dissection. Laryngoscope. 2007 May;117(5):797-802.

Folz BJ, Ferlito A, Silver CE, Olofsson J, Bradley PJ, Bieñ S, Towpik E, Weir N, Rinaldo A. Neck dissection in the nineteenth century. Eur Arch Otorhinolaryngol. 2007 May;264(5):455-60

Folz BJ, Silver CE, Rinaldo A, Fagan JJ, Pratt LW, Weir N, Seitz D, Ferlito A. An outline of the history of head and neck oncology. Oral Oncol. 2008 Jan;44(1):2-9.

Harvey, William. On the Motion of the Heart and Blood in Animals. London: George Bell and Sons 1889.

Jawdyn´ ski F. Przypadek raka pierwotnego szyi. t.z. raka skrzelowego Volkmann'a. Wycie˛ cie nowotworu wraz z rezekcyja˛ te˛ tnicy szyjowej wspo´ lnej i z˙ yły szyjowej wewne˛ trznej. Wyzdrowienie. Gaz Lek 1888;8:530–7.

Kocher T. Ueber Radicalheilung des Krebses. Dtsch Z Chir 1880;13:134–66.

Langenbeck B. Totalextirpation des Kehlkopfes mit dem Zungenbein, einem Theil der Zunge, des Pharynx und Oesophagus. Berl Klin Wschr 1875;12:33.

Leemans CR, Tiwari R, Nauta JJ, et al. Regional lymph node involvement and its significance in the development of distant metastases in head and neck carcinoma. Cancer 1993;71:452 - 6.

Leemans CR, Tiwari R, Nauta JJ, et al. Recurrence at the primary site in head and neck cancer and the significance of neck lymph node metastases as a prognostic factor. Cancer 1994;73:187 - 90.

Lister BJ. On the antiseptic principle in the practice of surgery. 1867. Clin Orthop Relat Res. 2010 Aug;468(8):2012-6.

Major RH. A history of medicine. Vol II. Thomas, SpringWeld; 1954: pp 752–754
Martin HE, Del Valle B, Ehrlich H, Cahan WG. Neck dissection. Cancer 1951;4:441–99.
Mendenhall WM, Parsons JT, Buatti JM, Stringer SP, Million RR, Cassisi NJ. Advances in radiotherapy for head and neck cancer. Semin Surg Oncol 1995;11:256–64.
Patel KN, Shah JP. Neck dissection: past, present, future. Surg Oncol Clin N Am 2005;14:461–77.
Rinaldo A, Ferlito A, Silver CE. Early history of neck dissection. Eur Arch Otorhinolaryngol. 2008; 265:1535–1538.
Robbins KT, Medina JE, Wolfe GT, Levine PA, Sessions RB, Pruet CW. Standardizing neck dissection terminology. Official report of the Academy's Committee for head and neck surgery and oncology. Arch Otolaryngol Head Neck Surg 1991;117:601–5.
Robbins KT, Clayman G, Levine P, Medina J, Sessions R, Shaha A, et al. Neck dissection classification update. Revisions proposed by the American Head and Neck Society and the American Academy of Otolaryngology—Head and Neck Surgery. Arch Otolaryngol Head Neck Surg 2002;128:751–8.
Robbins KT, Ferlito A, Sua´ rez C, Brizel DM, Bradley PJ, Pellitteri PK, et al. Is there a role for selective neck dissection after chemor- adiation for head and neck cancer? J Am Coll Surg 2004;199:913–6.
Robbins KT, Doweck I, Samant S, Vieira F. Effectiveness of super- selective and selective neck dissection for advanced nodal metastases after chemoradiation. Arch Otolaryngol Head Neck Surg 2005; 131:965–9.
Robbins KT, Shaha AR, Medina JE, Califano JA, Wolf GT, Ferlito A, Som PM, Day TA. Consensus statement on the classification and terminology of neck dissection. Arch Otolaryngol Head Neck Surg. 2008 May;134(5):536-8.
Shah JP, Strong E, Spiro RH, Vikram B. Neck dissection: current status and future possibilities. Clin Bull 1981;11:25–33.
Spiro JD, Spiro RH, Shah JP, Sessions RB, Strong EW. Critical assessment of supraomohyoid neck dissection. Am J Surg. 1988 Oct;156(4): 286-289.
Shapin S. The Scientific Revolution. Chicago: Univ. of Chicago Pr. 1996.
Suarez O. Distant and lymphatic metastases of cancer of the larynx and hypopharynx. Rev Otorrinolaringol 1963;23:83–99.
Sudhoff, Karl. Essays in the History of Medicine. Medical Life Press, New York 1926; 67-104.
Towpik E. Centennial of the first description of the en bloc neck dissection. Plast Reconstr Surg 1990;85:468–70.
Uttley AR, McGurk M. Sir Henry Trentham Butlin: the father of British head and neck surgery. Br J Oral Maxillofac Surg. 2000 Apr;38(2):114-20.
Vesalius A. De Humani Corporis Fabrica. 1543. On the Fabric of the Human Body, translated by W. F. Richardson and J. B. Carman. 5 vols. San Francisco and Novato: Norman Publishing, 1998-2009.
Virchow, RLK. Cellular Pathology as Based upon Physiological and Pathological Histology. London: John Churchill, 1860.
Warren JC. Surgical Observations on Tumours, with Cases and Operations. Boston: Crocker and Brewster; 1837.
Website. http://www.aboutcancer.com/neck_nodes_level.gif.

Wolf et al. Induction chemotherapy plus radiation compared with surgery plus radiation in patients with advanced laryngeal cancer. The Department of Veterans Affairs Laryngeal Cancer Study Group. N Engl J Med. Jun 1991;324(24):1685-90.

Part 2

Different Techniques of Neck Dissection & Complications

2

Neck Dissection – Techniques and Complications

Jaimanti Bakshi[1], Naresh K. Panda[2],
Abdul Wadood Mohammed[3] and Anil K. Dash[4]
[1]*Dept. Of Otolaryngology&HNS, PGIMER, CHANDIGRH*
[2]*Dept. Of Otolaryngology&HNS, PGIMER, CHANDIGARH*
[3]*Dept. Of Otolaryngology&HNS, PGIMER*
[4]*Dept. Of Otolaryngology&HNS, PGIMER, CHANDIGARH*
India

1. Introduction

"Neck dissection" refers to the surgical procedure where the lymphatics and the fibro fatty tissue of neck are removed as a treatment for cervical lymphatic metastasis. As malignancies of the upper aero-digestive tract mainly metastasize to the cervical lymph nodes, neck dissections are performed along with surgical excision of these malignancies.

2. Relevant anatomy

The cervical lymph nodes are surgically divided into six levels. Each level of lymph node is interconnected by lymphatic channels and drain specific anatomic sites of the aero-digestive tract.

Level 1a - sub-mental group

It is the midline group bounded on both sides by the anterior belly of digastrics and the hyoid bone inferiorly. Tumors of floor of mouth, anterior oral tongue, anterior mandibular alveolar ridge, and lower lip metastasize to these nodes.

Level 1b - submandibular group

These are the lymph node groups bounded by the anterior and posterior belly of digastric and mandible superiorly. The submandibular gland is usually included in the specimen when this group of lymph nodes is removed. Cancers of oral cavity, anterior nasal cavity, soft tissue structures of mid face and submandibular gland commonly metastasize to this group of lymph nodes.

Level 2a and 2b - upper jugular group

This group of lymph nodes is related to the upper $1/3^{rd}$ of the internal jugular vein. They are bounded by the skull base above , inferior border of hyoid bone below , lateral border of sternohyoid and stylohyoid anteriorly and posterior border of sternocleidomastoid posteriorly. This group is further divided by the vertical plane in relation to the spinal accessory nerve. Level 2a is anterior to this plane and level 2b is posterior. Cancers of oral cavity, nasal cavity, nasopharynx, oropharynx, hypopharynx, larynx and parotid gland mainly metastasize to this group.

Level 3 - middle jugular group

These lymph nodes are related to the middle 1/3rd of the internal jugular vein. This level is bounded by inferior border of hyoid bone above, inferior border of cricoid cartilage below, lateral border of sternohyoid anteriorly and posterior border of sternocleidomastoid posteriorly. Cancers of oral cavity, nasopharynx, oropharynx , hypopharynx, and larynx metastasize to this group of lymph nodes.

Level 4 - lower jugular group

This group of lymph nodes is related to the lower 1/3rd of internal jugular vein. They are bounded by the lateral border of sternohyoid anteriorly, posterior border of sternocleidomastoid posteriorly, inferior border of cricoid cartilage superiorly and the clavicle inferiorly. Cancers from hypopharynx, cervical esophagus and larynx metastasize to this level.

Level 5a and 5b - posterior triangle group

This group of lymph nodes is related to the lower 1/3rd of the internal jugular vein along the lower half of the spinal accessory nerve and the transverse cervical artery. They also included the supraclavicular group of nodes. They are bounded by the posterior border of sternocleidomastoid anteriorly, anterior border of trapezius posteriorly and inferiorly the clavicle. Sublevel 5a and 5b are separated by a horizontal plane marking the inferior border of arch of the cricoid cartilage. Cancers of the nasopharynx, oropharynx and the thyroid gland mainly metastasize to this group.

Level 6 - anterior compartment group

This group includes the pre and para tracheal nodes, the precricoid (Delphian) and the perithyroidal nodes. They are bounded by hyoid bone superiorly, supra sternal notch inferiorly and common carotid arteries laterally. Cancers arising from the thyroid gland, glottic and subglottic larynx, apex of pyriform sinus and cervical esophagus mainly metastasize to this group of lymph nodes.

3. History

- In 1888, ***Jawdynski*** described en bloc resection of cervical lymph nodes with resection of carotid, internal jugular vein and sternocleidomastoid muscle which was associated with very high rate of mortality.
- In 1906, ***George W. Crile*** of the Cleveland Clinic described the radical neck dissection. The operation encompasses removal of all the lymph nodes on one side along with the spinal accessory nerve, internal jugular vein and sternocleidomastoid muscle.
- In 1967 - ***Oscar Suarez*** and ***E. Bocca*** described a more conservative operation which preserves spinal accessory nerve, internal jugular vein and sternocleidomastoid muscle which further improved the quality of life of patients post operatively.

4. Classification of neck dissections

The classification proposed by the Committee for head and neck surgery and oncology of the American Academy of Otolaryngology and Head and Neck surgery is the first comprehensive classification widely accepted. It is based on the rationale that radical neck dissection is the standard basic procedure for cervical lymphadenectomy, and all other procedures represent one or more modifications of this procedure. When the modification of the radical neck dissection involves *preservation* of one or more *non-lymphatic structures,* the procedure is termed a modified radical neck dissection, when the modification involves *preservation* of one or more *lymph node groups* that are routinely removed in the radical neck dissection; the procedure is termed a selective neck dissection and when the modification involves removal of *additional lymph node groups or non-lymphatic structures* relative to the radical neck dissection, the procedure is termed an extended radical neck dissection.

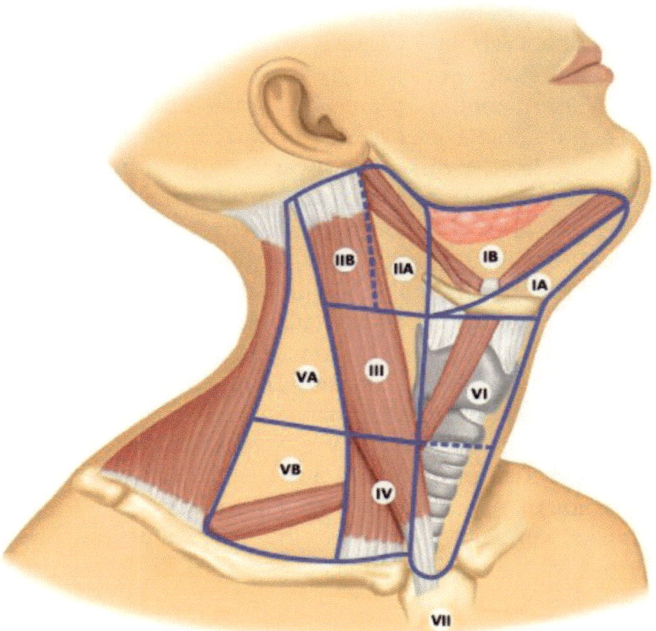

Fig. 1. Lymph node levels of neck

Medina et al has suggested that the term"comprehensive neck dissection" be used whenever all of the lymph nodes contained in levels I through V have been removed. Hence, the radical neck dissection and modified radical neck dissection would each be considered a comprehensive neck dissection.

Three subtypes of modified radical neck dissection were recommended to denote which of the three non lymphatic structures were removed. The neck dissection is labeled as type 1, when only spinal accessory nerve is preserved, type 2 when spinal accessory nerve and the internal jugular vein was preserved and type 3 when all three non lymphatic structures were preserved. Spiro et al also have suggested changes to the existing Academy's classification system. He used the term radical neck dissection when 4 or 5 levels are resected, which included conventional radical neck dissection, modified radical neck dissection and extended radical neck dissection. The term selective neck dissection was used when 3 levels of lymph nodes are dissected and limited neck dissection when no more than 2 levels of lymph nodes are dissected.

Surgical procedure:

Radical Neck Dissection: Procedure is done under general anesthesia. Position the patient in reverse Trendelenberg's position with neck extended at atlanto-axial joint and head elevated 10 degree above the table. Face should be turned to the opposite side of the dissection. Neck skin should be cleaned with Betadine scrub and after that with 3 layers of Betadine solution. Drap the operating site with sterile towels over a polydrape sheet to minimize the infection rate. Our preferred incision for R.N.D. is Lahey's lateral utility incision in post-irradiated patients. Modified Schobinger's incision has been found to be useful in patients undergoing commando operation. We are using Mc fees double horizontal incision in some selected post-irradiated cases.

Incision is marked with surgical marker pen, infiltrate with 10-15 ml of 1% xylocaine with 1:4 lacs adrenaline solution. Wait for 5 minutes , make skin incision with 10 number surgical blade, raise the sub-platysmal flap superiorly till lower border of mandible, mastoid tip posteriorly, midline of neck anteriorly, anterior border of trapezius posteriorly, and till clavicle inferiorly. Then the lower part of sterno-cliedomastiod muscle is cut with electro-cautery, 2cms above clavicle after dissecting it carefully from internal jugular vein. Dissect the IJV from its fascial attachments with common carotid artery and vagus nerve. The lower end of IJV is ligated at level of common tendinous attachment of 2 bellies of omo-hyoid muscle crossing over IJV. Transfix the IJV after ligating with double ligatures. Pull the IJV up gradually with SCM muscle after holding with Babcock forceps. Dissect all lymph nodes, lymphatics,fat and fascia from the supra clavicular fossa including level 5 nodes. Take care not to damage the brachial plexus, phrenic nerve, transverse cervical vessels. At the junction of upper 1/3 and lower 2/3 of SCM muscle, greater auricular nerve,can be seen exiting from cervical plexus crossing over external jugular vein along posterior border. GAN winds around the posterior border of SCM muscle and crosses obliquely upwards to enter into the tail of parotid gland. Spinal accessory nerve also exits at this point, known as Erb's point and runs in the posterior triangle to enter into trapezius muscle. These nerves have to be dissected from cutaneous branches supplying the fascia and skin. Ligate middle thyroid vein at level of thyroid cartilage and remove all lymph nodes along the middle 1/3 of IJV thus clearing level 3&4. Now, we have reached at the upper end of IJV. Dissect at the level of posterior belly of digastric muscle which is the landmark for ligating the upper end. Bony landmark is the transverse process of atlas. Ligate with double ligatures, transfix with 3-0 silk suture and cut the IJV after ligating the venae commitante for hypoglossal nerve. This will clear level 2a & 2b lymph nodes. Last step is removal of level 1a & 1b nodes along with submandibular gland. Remove the complete specimen enbloc. Irrigate the dissected field with normal saline and dilute betadine solution. After securing hemostasis, put Romovac 14-16 FG size drain, fix it with braided silk sutures, and connect to the bellow. After repositing the skin flap, first layer is sutured with 3-0 vicryl/ catgut suture and skin with staples /3-0 Ethicon monocryl sutures. Apply pressure dressing and check the drain function before extubating the patient. Post opetatively, patient is kept in fowler's position and give I.V. antibiotics for 5 days. Remove drain when collection is < 10 ml. Remove sutures on 7th post operative day. Discharge the patient on 7th day. Follow up will be after 1 week, check the histopathology report to see how many lymph nodes were dissected and the number of positive nodes. Refer for radiotherapy if needed. Thereafter at 1 month. Contrast CT scan /PET-CT scan should be ordered at 6 month follow up for recurrent disease. One monthly follow up will continue for 1 year ,thereafter 3 monthly for 2 years and then yearly for 10 years.

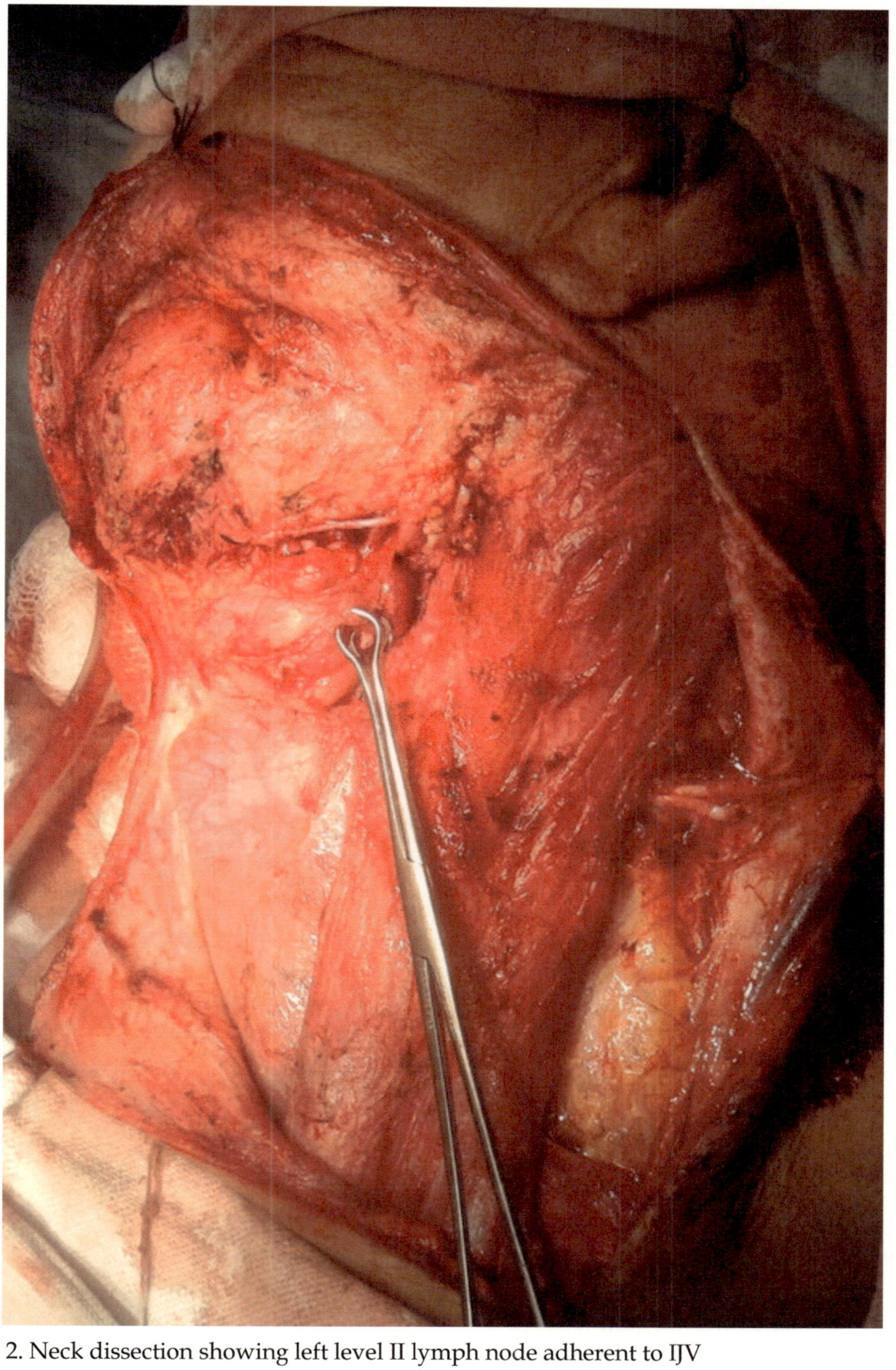

Fig. 2. Neck dissection showing left level II lymph node adherent to IJV

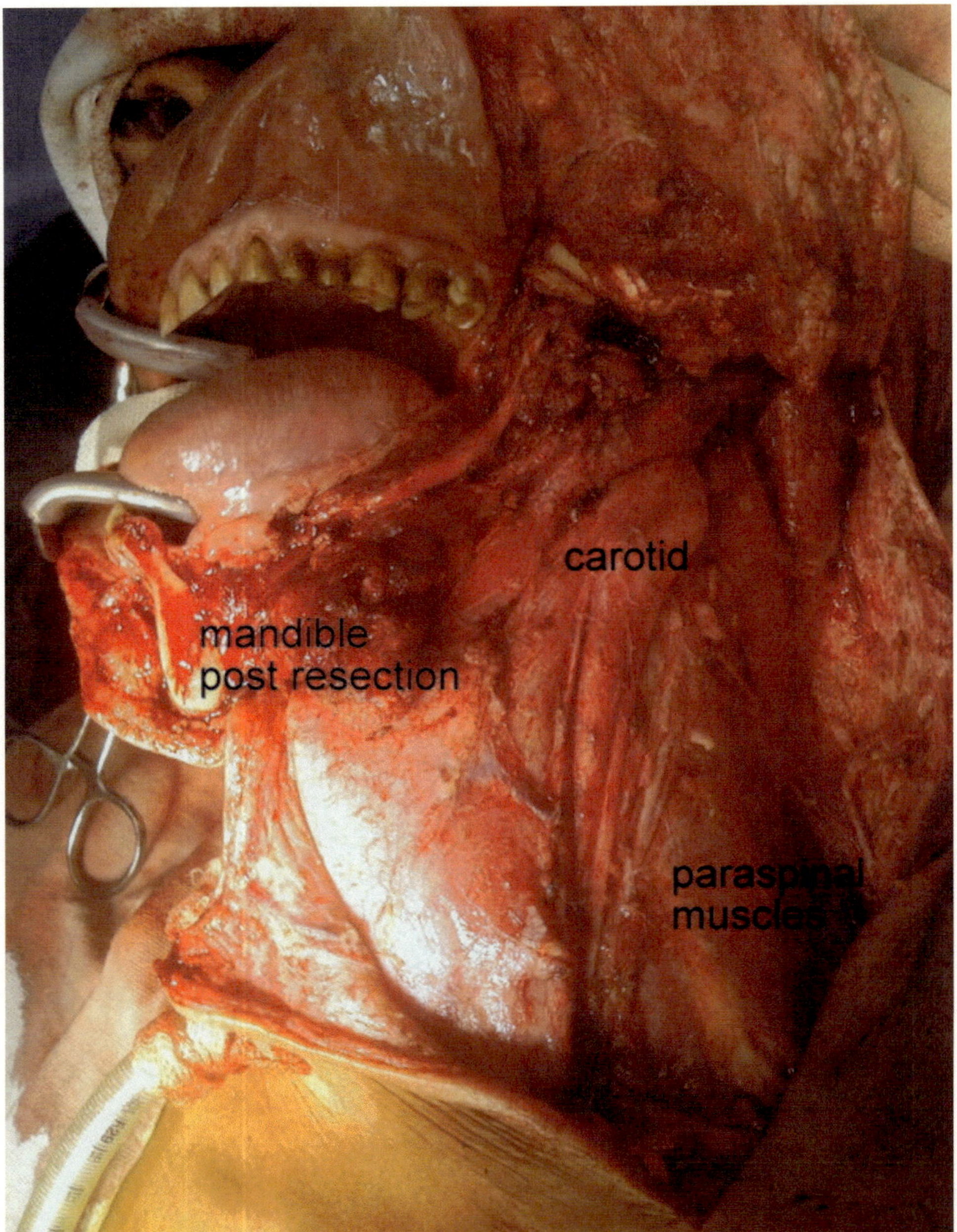

Fig. 3. Commando operation showing left radical neck dissection

Modified Neck Dissection:

The basic procedure will remain same as for RND but we have to preserve one/more than one of the 3 structures i.e. SCM muscle, Spinal accessory nerve and IJV. Preserve the greater auricular nerve and transverse cervical vessels for decreased morbidity.

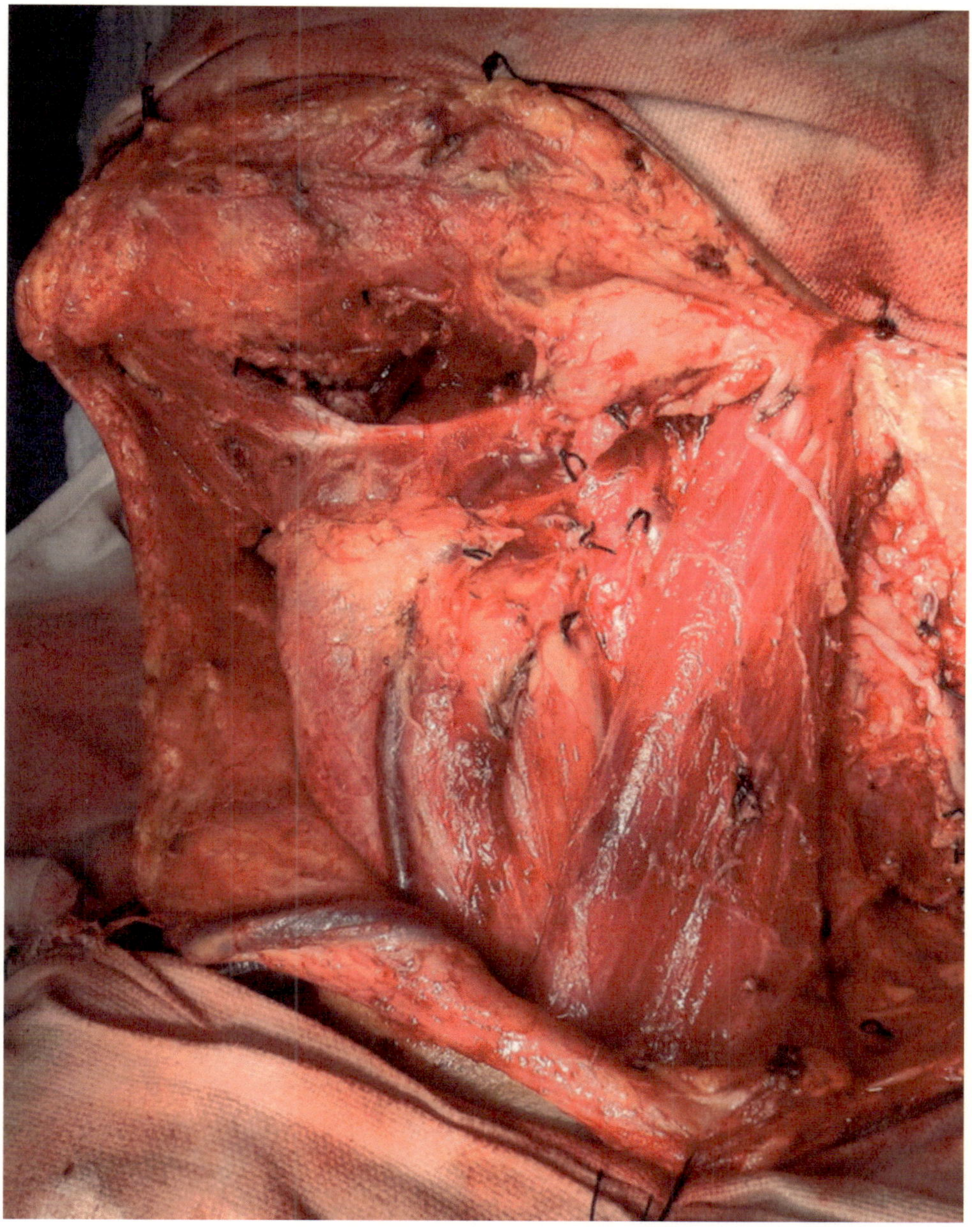

Fig. 4. Post Modified Radical Neck Dissection on Left side

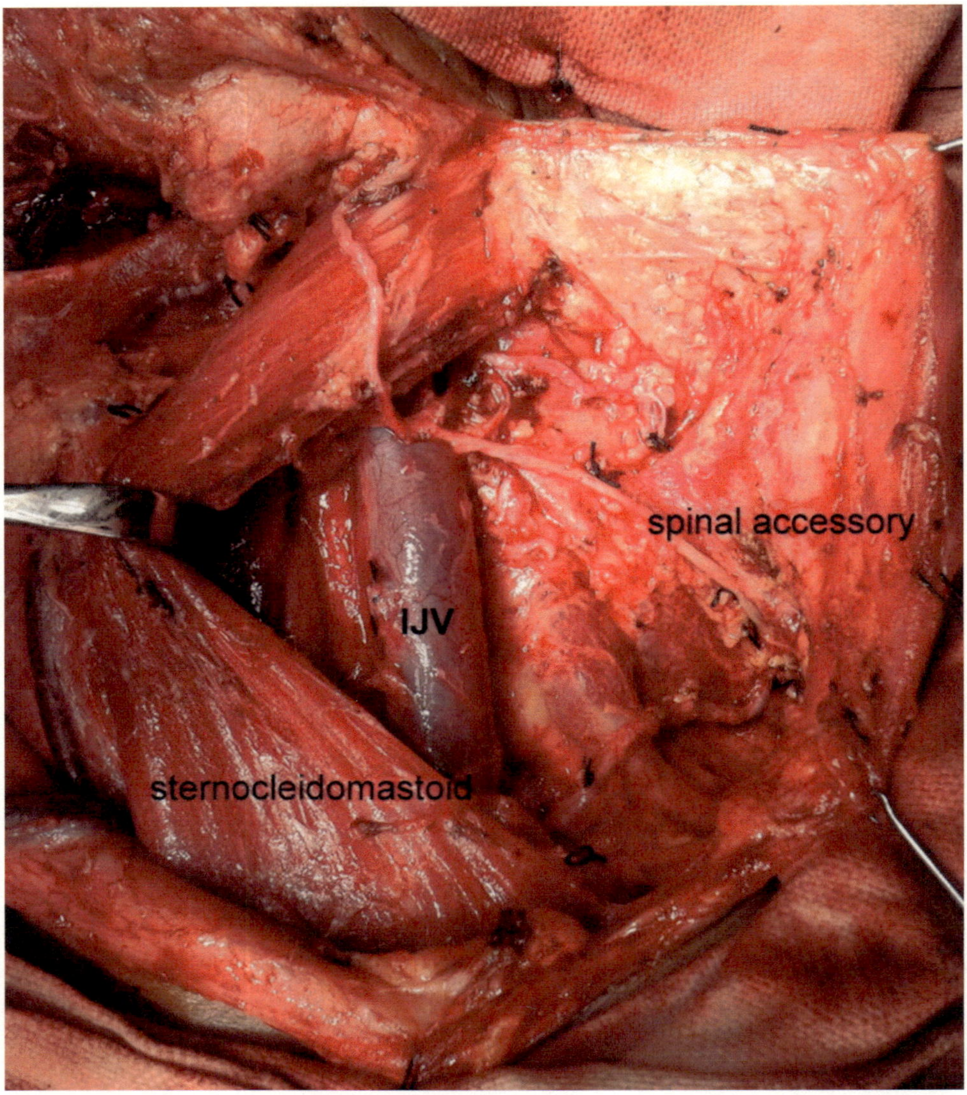

Fig. 5. Left Modified Radical Neck dissection exposing preserved structures

Selective Neck Dissection:

Modified Schobinger incision/ Apron flap incision are the best incisions for this procedure. Dissection will start from level I and will go to level III/IV in Supra omohyoid neck dissection and will include level VI in Anterior compartment dissection.

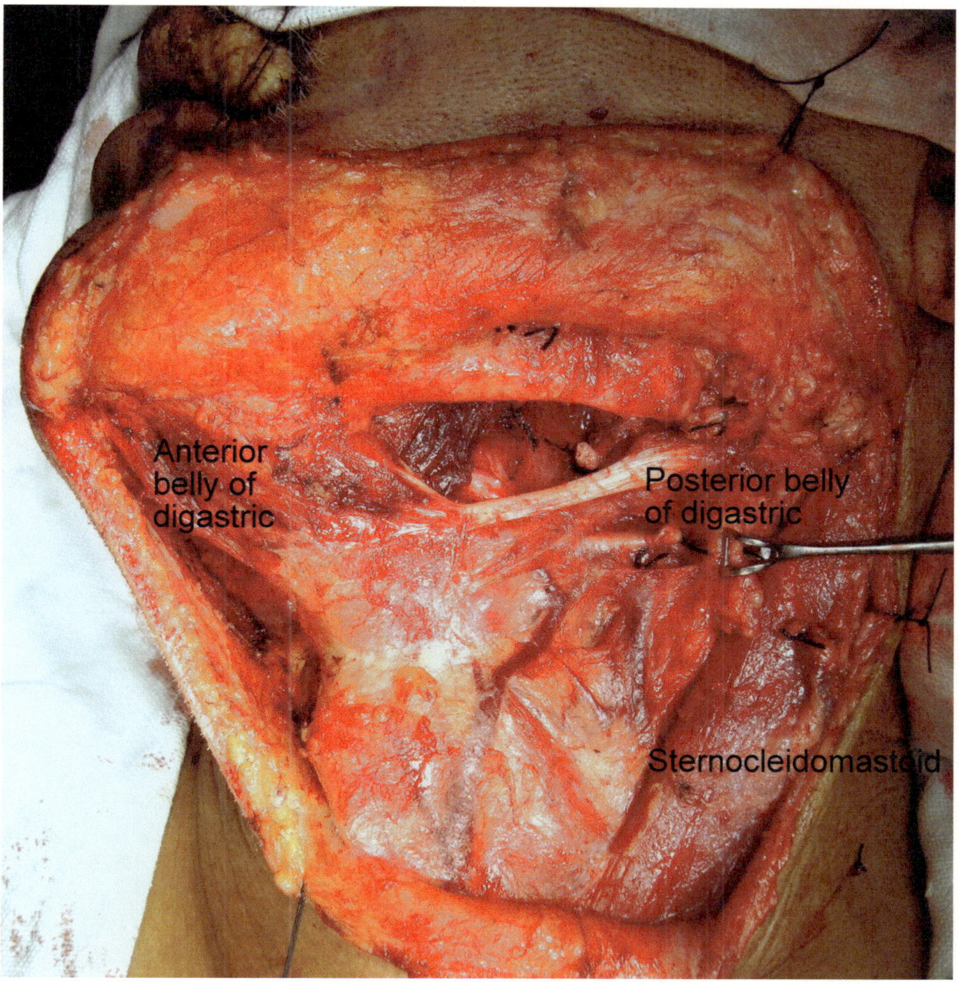

Fig. 6. Post left supra-omohyoid neck dissection

5. Our experience

Type 3 Modified neck dissections and selective neck dissections are the most common neck dissections performed in our institute. The decision is made intra operatively. In general,for N0 neck , supraomohyoid neck dissection and for N1 neck, type 3 modified radical neck dissection is done. Radical neck dissection is done only when there is gross infilteration of the sternocleidomastoid muscle or spinal accessory nerve or internal jugular vein intra operatively or in post irradiated neck.

Modified schobinger's incision is the most common incision used for Modified radical neck dissection. It has the advantage of adequate exposure and the incision can be easily extended anteriorly as lip splitting incision in order to expose the primary oral cavity tumor. The Lahey's lateral utility incision is commonly used in post irradiated neck as it has the advantage of not forming a three point junction and prevents wound dehiscence and carotid blow out. Transverse cervical neck incision would suffice for supra omohyoid neck dissection. Other incisions occasionally used are the Wisor flap, Boomerang incision and Mc fee's incision. Post operatively negative suction drains are put for an average period of 3-5 days and patient needs hospital admission for an average period of 10 days. Plan for post operative radiotherapy is done according to the stage of disease and post operative histopathology report. External Beam radiotherapy is given in the dose of 50 to 55 Grays in 20 to 30 fractions with in a period of 6 weeks started as early as possible when the wound is healed. Radiotherapy is given for all advanced stage disease (Stage 3 and 4) and when the histopathology report shows resection margins involved or close to tumour, more than 2 lymph nodes involved, perineural spread or extracapsular spread.
Figures 7, 8, 9 show the types of incisions which we use for neck dissections.

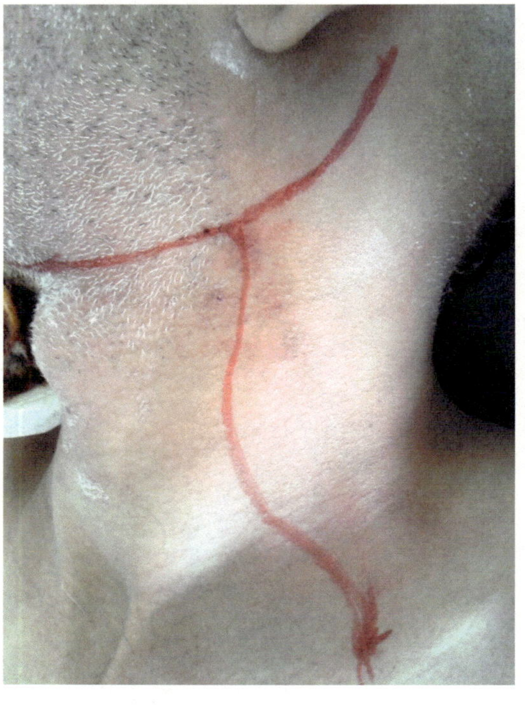

Fig. 7. Modified Schobinger's incision

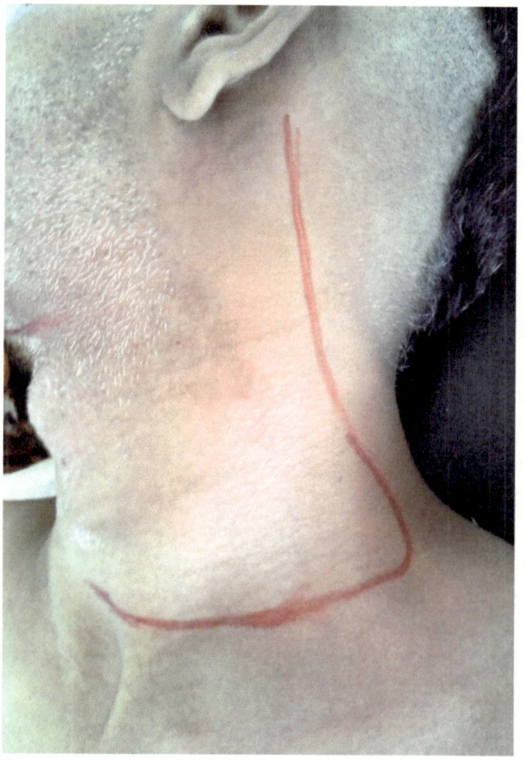

Fig. 8. Lateral Utility incision Lahey's

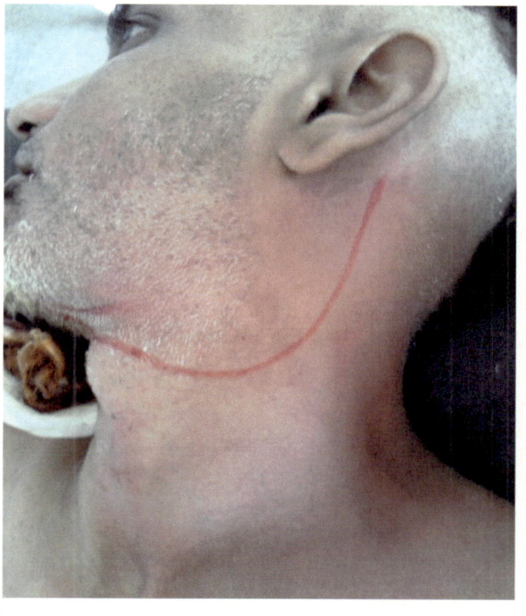

Fig. 9. Apron flap incision

6. Complications

1. Anesthesia of the skin of the neck is most common complication.
2. Black/ bluish discoloration of the skin flap at 3 point junction or at posterior lip can occur in some patients.
3. Minor wound dehiscences and wound infections can occur in some.
4. Seroma formation has been seen occasionally.
5. Chyle leak can occur in 2-3% patients and heals with conservative treatment most of the times. No patient required neck exploration for repair of the thoracic duct.
6. Air embolism can occur in <1% cases due to inadvertent injury to IJV.
7. Carotid blow out has been seen in < 1% patients after RND. It is common in irradiated necks

Case 1

32 year old male presented to our out patient department with complaints of non healing ulcer over the tongue for which he was taking medication from local practisioners. He had been taking Gutka (a local tobacco preparation) and was smoking cigarettes around cigarattes 2 - 3 packs/day for 15 years. On examination he had a 2 x 2 cm ulcero indurated lesion over the right lateral border of tongue. His neck examination showed a 1 x 1.5 cm right level 1b lymph node. A PET/CT was done for metastatic work up which showed intense uptake over the lesion on the right lateral border of tongue, moderate uptake in right level 1b and 2 lymph nodes and no distant metastasis. Patient underwent right partial glossectomy with right type 3 functional neck dissection. The post operative histopathology report came as all resection margins free of tumor, however the posterior resection margin was close to tumor and 0/33 lymph nodes free of tumor. Patient underwent post operative external radiotherapy of 55 Gys 25 fractions in 6 weeks and is now on follow up for the last 6 months without any locoregional recurrence.

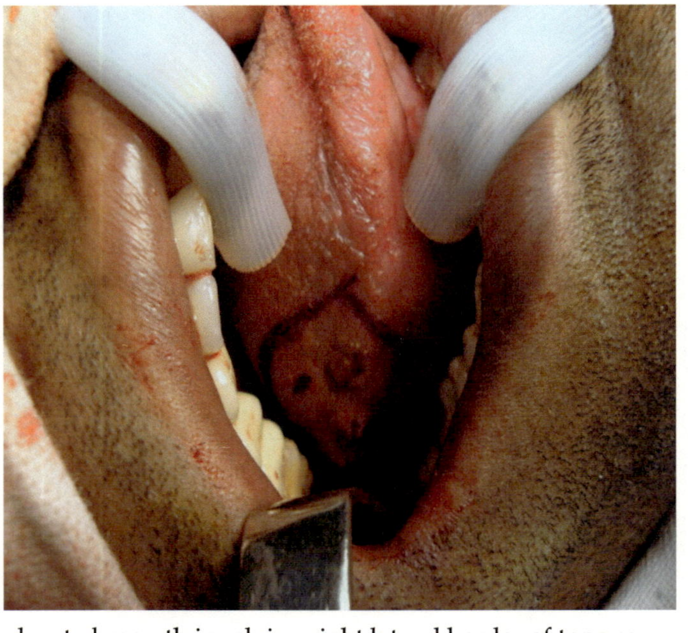

Fig. 10. Ulcero indurated growth involving right lateral border of tongue

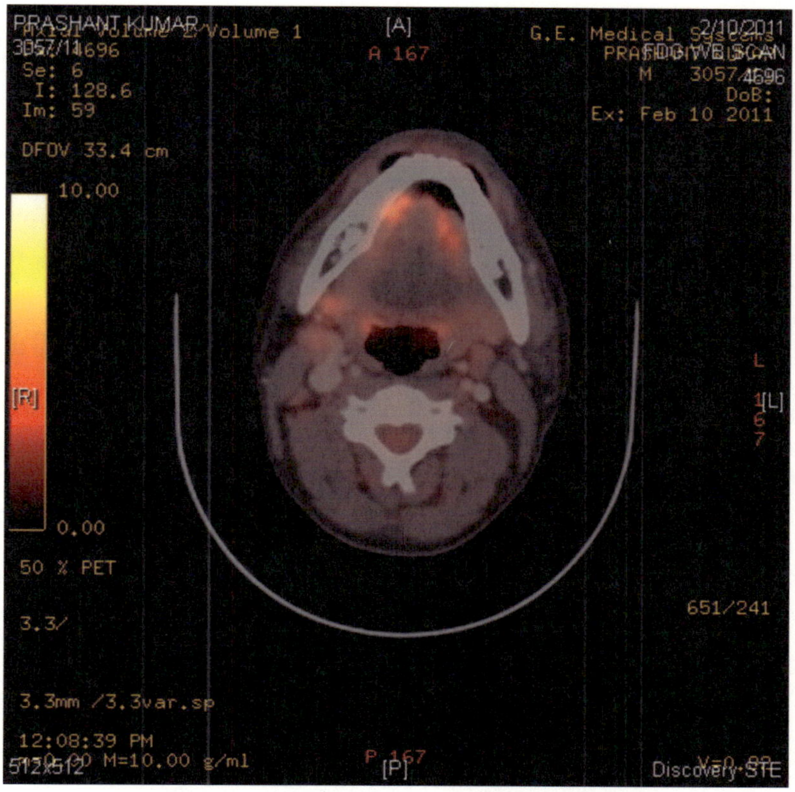

Fig. 11. PET/CT showing increased uptake in right lateral border of tongue and Right level 1b and 2 lymph nodes

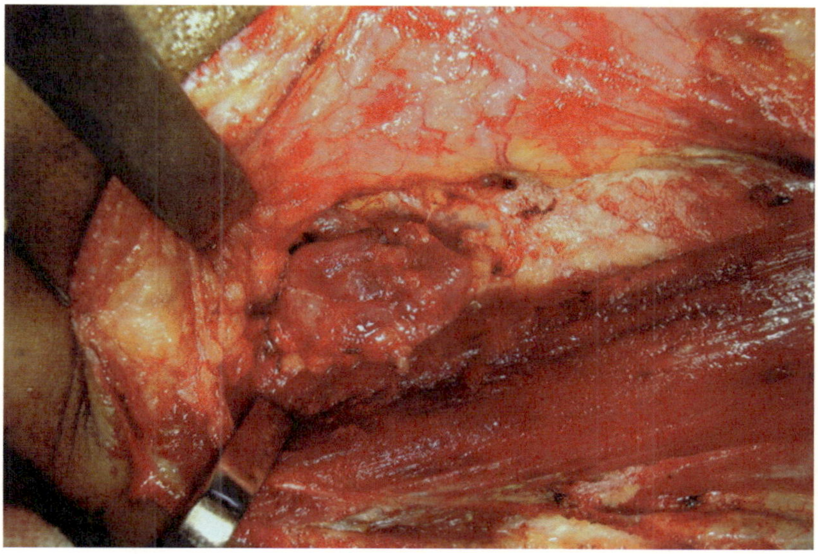

Fig. 12. Right level 1b lymph node

Case 2

50 year old chronic Zarda chewer (local tobacco preparation) and cigarette smoker presented with growth over the left lower alveolus for 3 months. On examination he had a 4 x 3 cm ulcero proliferative growth extending from the (L) lateral incisor to the 3 rd molar involving the lower gingivo buccal sulcus and the buccal mucosa till the level of crown of teeth. There was a 3x 3 cm swelling over the left mandible 1 cm away from the angle of mouth with free overlying skin. On neck examination the left level 1b had 1x 1 cm lymph node and level 2 3 x 2 cm. A PET/CT was done for metastatic work up which showed intense uptake SUV 22.3 over the lesion over (L) lower alveolus and (L) level 1b and 2 without any distant metastasis. Patient underwent (L) segmental mandibulectomy with (L) Radical neck dissection as the level 2 lymph node was adherent to the IJV and sternocleidomastoid intra operatively and reconstruction with pectoralis major myocutaneous flap. Patient received 50 Gys External Radiotherapy and is disease free for 12 months.

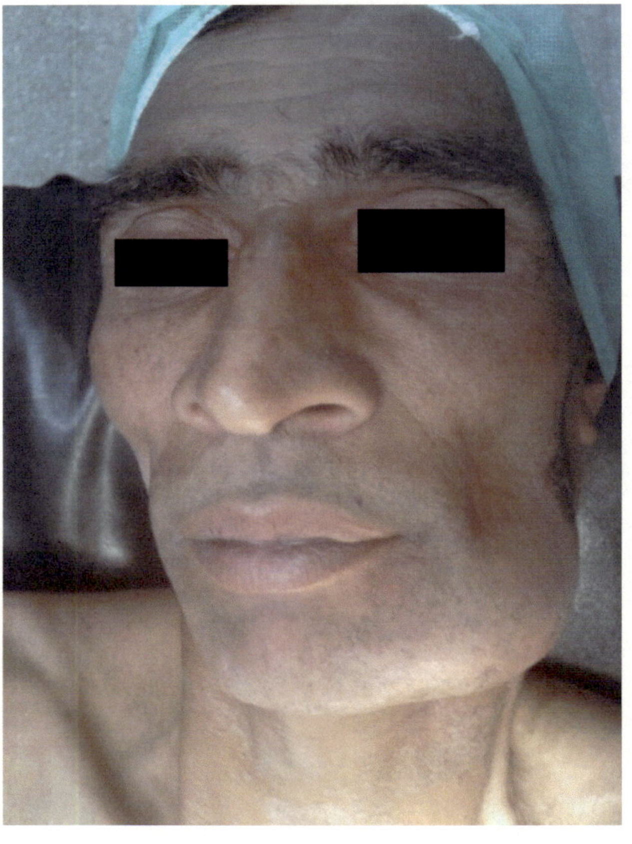

Fig. 13. case 2

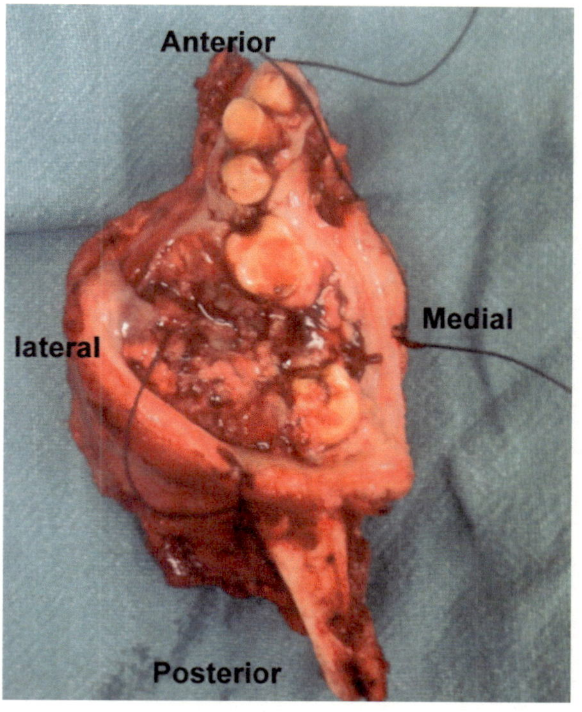

Fig. 14. Segmental mandibulectomy with tumor

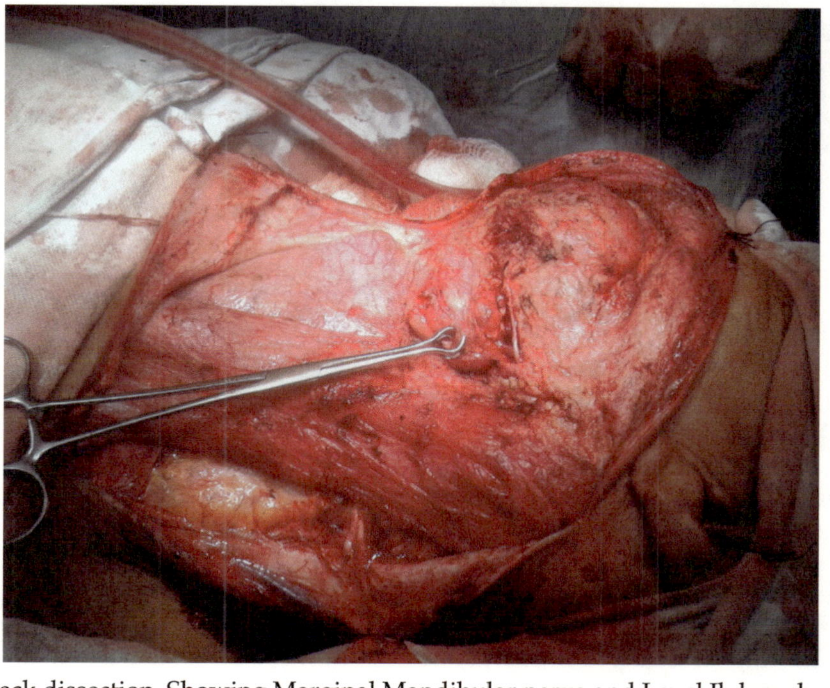

Fig. 15. Neck dissection. Showing Marginal Mandibular nerve and Level Ib lymph node

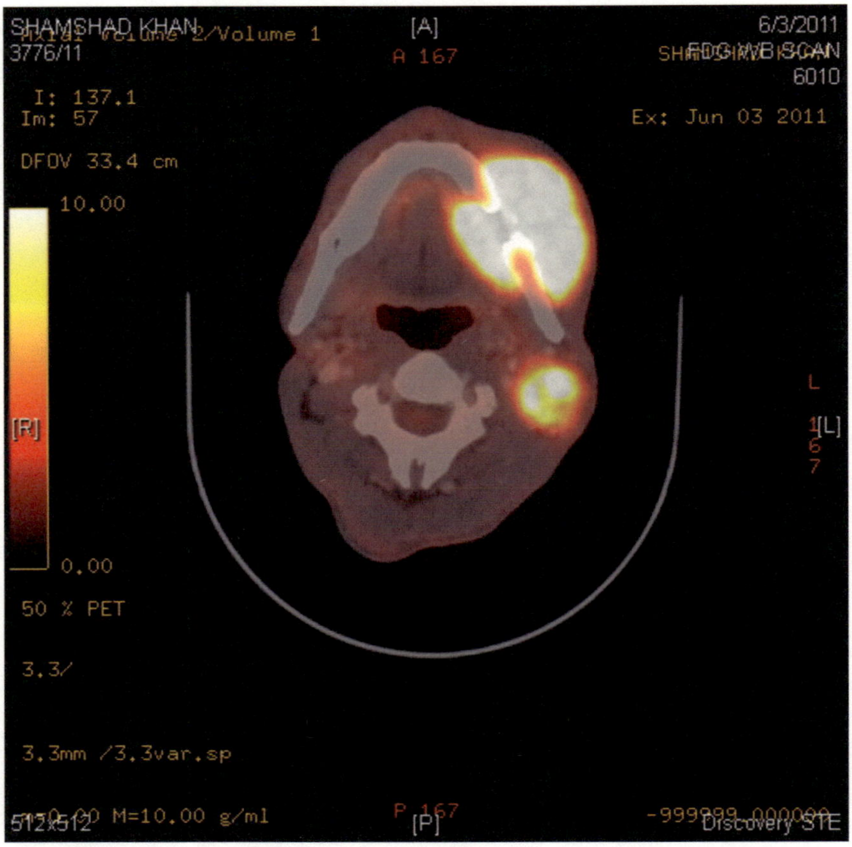

Fig. 16. PET/CT image case 2

Case 3

37 year old female with no history of any addiction presented with history of swelling over the left cheek which was rapidly increasing in size and difficulty in opening mouth for 3 month. On examination there was a 6 x 8 cm swelling over the left cheek which was fluctuant. The swelling late ruptured to form an ulcer as shown in figure 17. There was a 3 x 3 cm ulcer in the left buccal mucosa with extension into the lower gingivo buccal sulcus. On neck examination left level 1b was 1 x 2 cm enlarged. CECT of neck was done which showed the primary tumor involving left buccal mucosa and skin with ipsilateral involvement of level 1b and 2 lymph node levels. The patient underwent a Wide local excision with left type 3 modified neck dissection and the defect was reconstructed using antero-lateral thigh free flap. The patient received 60 Gys postoperative radiotherapy over 6 weeks and is disease free for 12 months now.

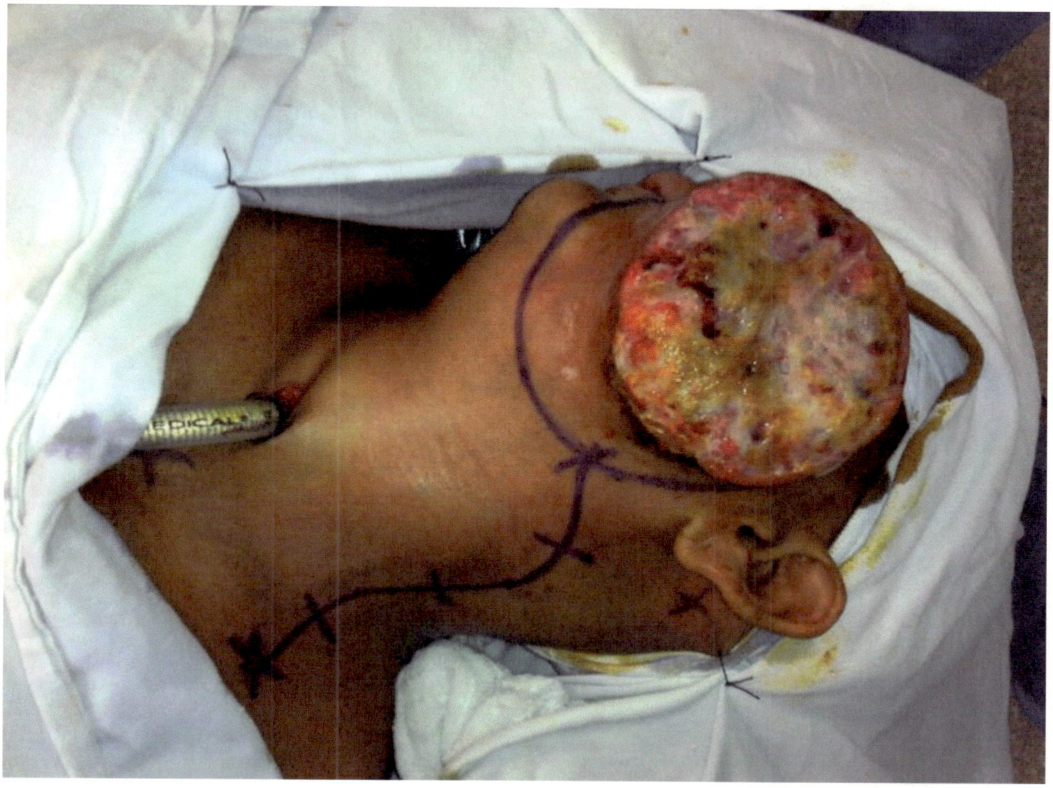

Fig. 17. Primary lesion. Incision is modified for resection of primary tumor

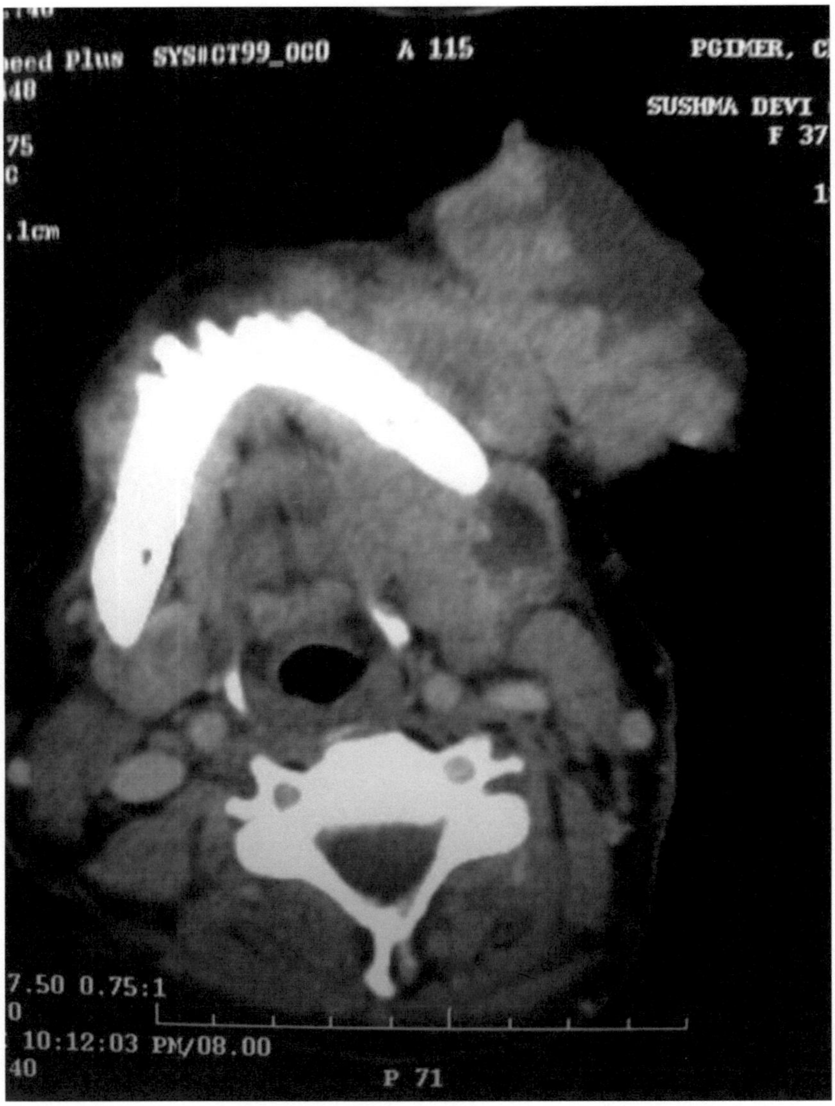

Fig. 18. CECT of case 3 showing primary tumour and neck node

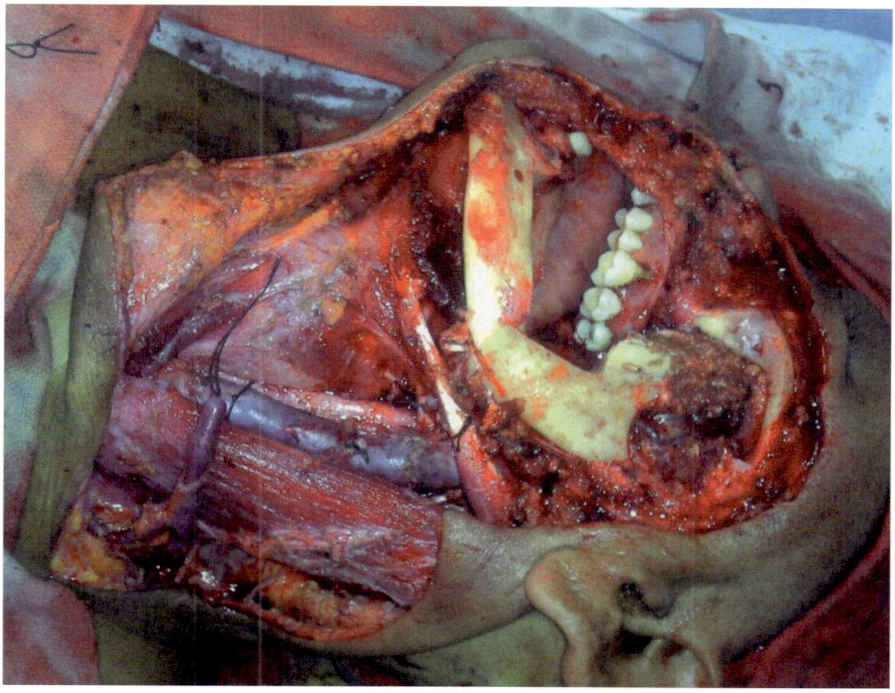

Fig. 19. Post resection with Segmental Mandibulectomy and Modified neck dissection

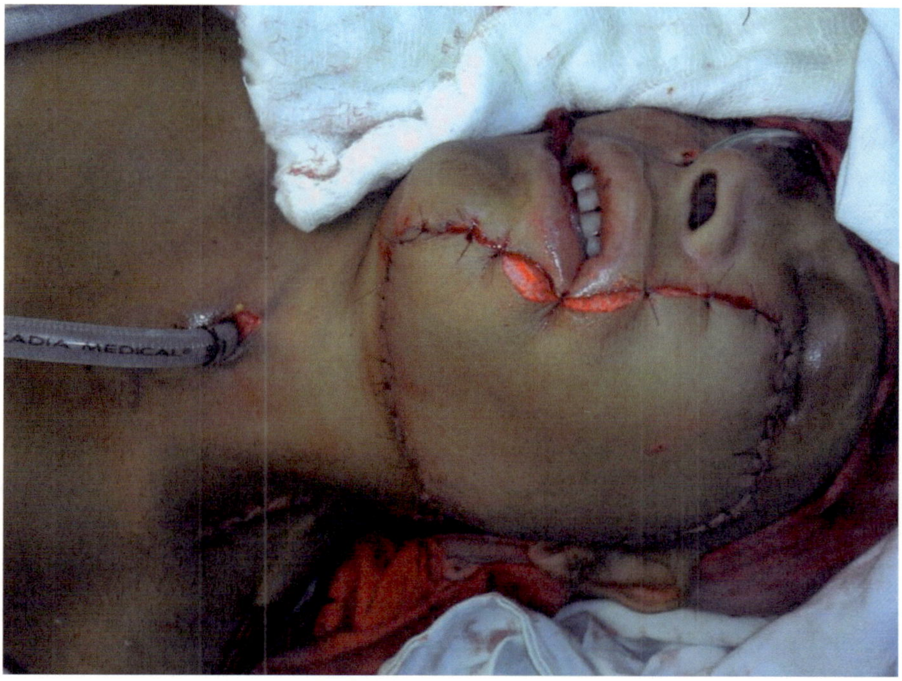

Fig. 20. After reconstruction with Antero lateral thigh free flap

Complications

Complications of neck dissection can be broadly divided into early, intermediate and late.

Immediate

Hemorrhage

Postoperative hemorrhage usually occurs immediately after surgery. External bleeding through the incision often originates in a subcutaneous blood vessel. In most patients, this may be readily controlled by ligation, direct cauterization or infiltration of the surrounding tissues with an anesthetic solution containing epinephrine. Pronounced swelling or ballooning of the skin flaps immediately after surgery, with or without external bleeding, should be attributed to a hematoma in the wound. If a hematoma is detected early, "milking" the drains occasionally may result in evacuation of the accumulated blood and the problem will resolve. If this is not accomplished immediately or if blood re-accumulates quickly, it is best to return the patient to the operating room, explore the wound under sterile conditions, evacuate the hematoma, and control the bleeding.

Airway obstruction

In cases of bilateral neck dissections there may be associated soft tissue edema. Moreover resection of the primary upper aero-digestive malignancy may also add to the edema of the airway. It is always prudent to carry out a temporary elective tracheotomy to protect the airway.

Increased intracranial pressure

This usually occurs when the internal jugular vein is ligated. When one internal jugular vein is ligated the pressure rises by 3 fold and when both are ligated it increases by 5 fold. This usually is temporary and will normalize in 24 hours. If it persists, head end elevation, steroids and mannitol can be used.

Nerve injury

The main nerves which are at risk during neck dissection are spinal accessory nerve, vagus nerve, hypoglossal nerve, phrenic nerve and lingual nerve. Spinal accessory nerve injury causes difficulty in shrugging shoulders and shoulder hand syndrome. Hypoglossal nerve injury will cause tongue paralysis. Vagus nerve injury may manifest as aspiration and voice problems. Phrenic nerve injury causes paradoxical breathing and lingual nerve injury causes taste problems. Neuropraxia may recover within months; where as neurotemesis and axonotemesis have varying outcome.

Carotid sinus syndrome

This is due to undue pressure and manipulation on the carotid sinus baroreceptor which may result in hypotension and bradycardia. Post operative scarring may also make the receptor sensitive to even palpation and turning head.

Pneumothorax

Too much lower neck dissection may cause injury to the apical pleura causing pneumothorax. Patient may become restless, cyanosed and dyspnoeic after operation. A plain radiograph of chest most often provides the diagnosis. Minimal emphysema may resolve itself but whereas severe cases may require intercostal chest drains.

Intermediate complications

Pulmonary complications

Basal collapse and bronchopneumonia may occur in patients who are smokers and have pre-existing chronic obstructive lung disease.

Deep vein thrombosis

This is seen in patients in old age, surgeries lasting for more duration, long bedridden patients and patients with previous history of deep vein thrombosis, pulmonary embolism, myocardial infarction and thrombophilia.

Chylous fistula

This happens due injury to the thoracic duct while performing a radical surgery low in the neck or mediastinum. If chylous fistula is suspected every attempt should be made to seal it at the time of surgery by identifying it by head down positions and performing modified valsalva manoeuvre. It should be suspected when the drain collection increases dramatically by volume. Fat restricted diet, and daily pressure dressings are the form of conservative treatment for chyle leak. When the drain collection reaches 600 ml per day or more, it is an indication for exploration and repair of the injured thoracic duct under microscope.

Carotid artery rupture

This usually occurs when the skin wound breaks down because of previous irradiation, secondary infection, poor metabolic condition of the patient. It is a fatal complication resulting in immediate mortality if not intervened immediately. Control of bleeding by immediate finger pressure, airway management, blood transfusion and exploration in operation theatre has to be done.

Late complications

Recurrence

Recurrences can be at the primary site, in the neck nodes or as a distant metastasis.

Lymph edema

When both the internal jugular veins are ligated , lymphedema often follows owing to interruption of the lymphatic drainage channels from the head.

Hypertrophic scars

Author's experience

From year 1998 to 2011, the author has done over 250 neck dissections which included around 50 selective neck dissections and 200 comprehensive neck dissections. Out of the 200 comprehensive neck dissections, 75 were radical neck dissections and 125 were modified neck dissections. However if we look at the year wise distribution, we could clearly see a change in trend from radical neck dissection to less radical, modified radical neck dissection. 60 out of 75 i.e. 91% were done before year 2006 and 15 ie only 9 % were done after 2006.
A separate study has been done in year 2009-2010 by Bakshi et al which compared selective neck dissection with modified/radical neck dissection in terms of outcome and disease control in patients with carcinoma of buccal mucosa and also analyzed whether selective neck dissection can be used as a safe and effective treatment modality in N0 and N+ necks in cases of carcinoma buccal mucosa. The study included 22 patients who underwent

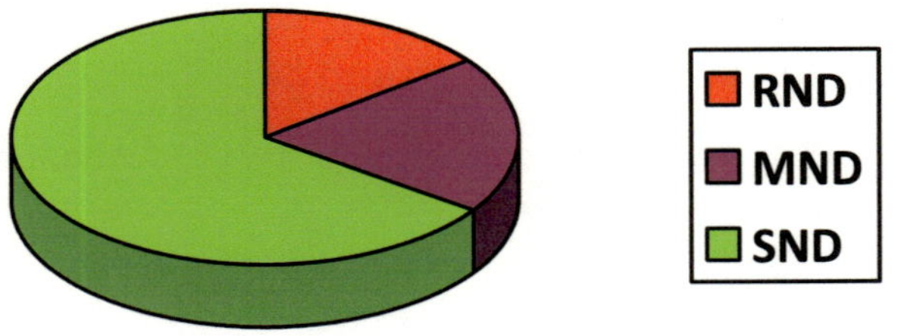

Fig. 21. Number of neck dissections by author

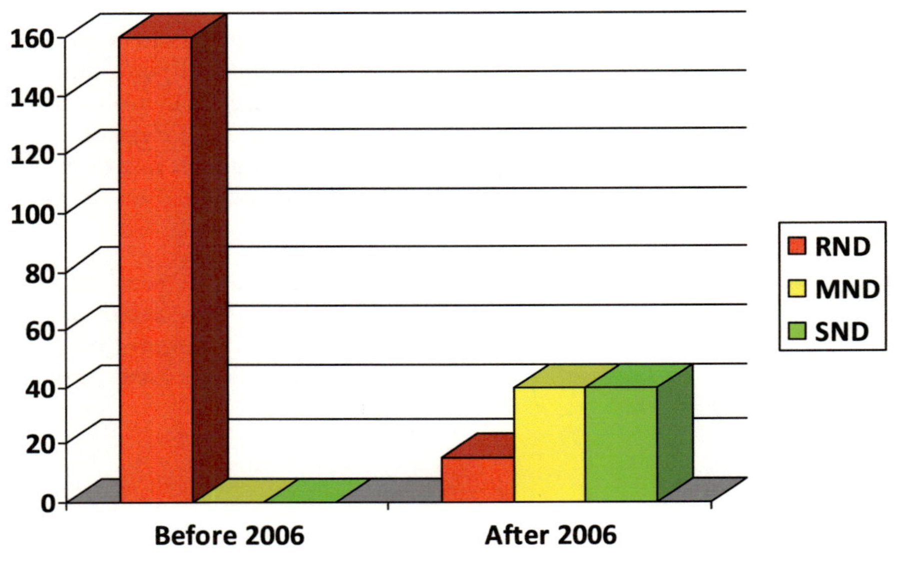

Fig. 22. Year wise distribution of Neck dissections

modified/radical neck dissection and 20 patients who underwent selective neck dissection. It was seen that 16(38.09%) patients out of the total group of 42 patients , had recurrence/residual disease at the time of completion of study whereas the remaining 26 patients(61.91%) were disease free for a minimum period of 6 months (ranging from 12-24months) with a mean follow up of 18 months . When studied group wise it was noticed that 9 (40.90%) patients in Group A (RADICAL NECK DISSECTION/MODIFIED RADICAL NECK DISSECTION) had recurrence whereas only 7 (35%) patients in Group B(SELECTIVE NECK DISSECTION) had recurrence. The difference between the number of patients with recurrent disease between the groups was not found to be statistically significant (p=0.790). The study puts into perspective, selective neck dissection in the cases of carcinoma buccal mucosa, as a safe and effective modality for addressing the neck disease in both N0 and N1, N2a and N2b necks with failure rate being comparable to that of radical/modified radical neck dissections. Hence patients can be spared from the morbidity of more radical procedures without compromising on the oncological safety. Most common lymphnode group involved in this study was level Ib followed by IIa.

Another study done by the author which analysed the outcome of surgical treatment for squamous cell carcinoma of the oral cavity taking into consideration mode of presentation, histopathological aspects, treatment , recurrence, prognostic factors and survival in patients undergoing various surgical modalities for primary oral cancer and metastatic cervical nodes. The study included 80 patients and was done between 2001 and 2006. The study concluded that combined modality of treatment would be a better approach to deal with advanced oral cancer as it offers good loco regional control and survival rate. However, tumor size and extent, type and grade, the neck node status and the status of excision margins do affect surgical prognosis and survival rate.

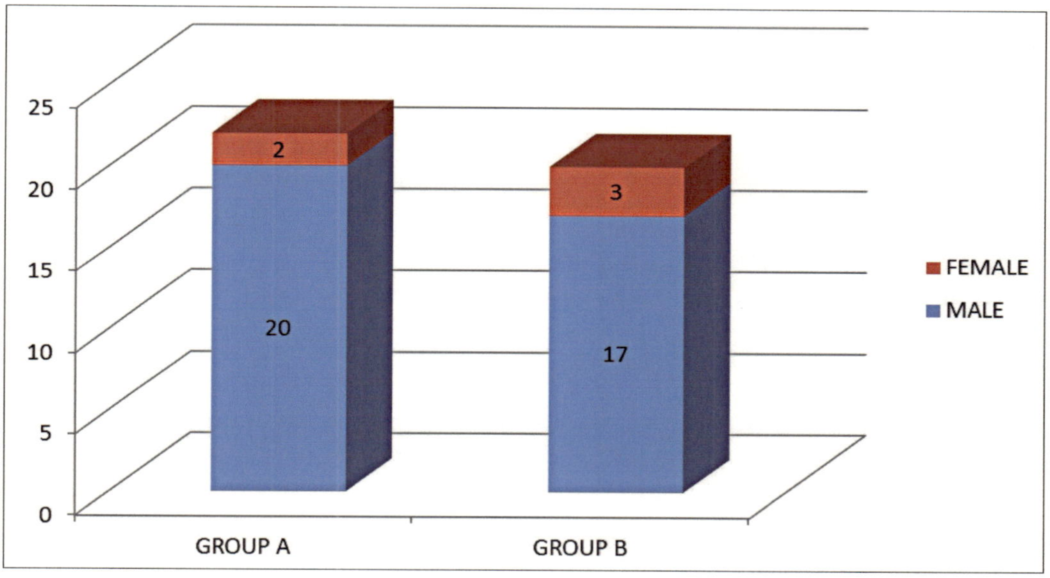

Fig. 23. Patient Distribution

			Group A	Group B	Total
OUTCOME	Recurrence	Count	9	7	16
		% within Group	40.9%	35.0%	38.09%
	Survived	Count	13	13	26
		% within Group	59.1%	65.0%	61.91%

Table 1. Study results

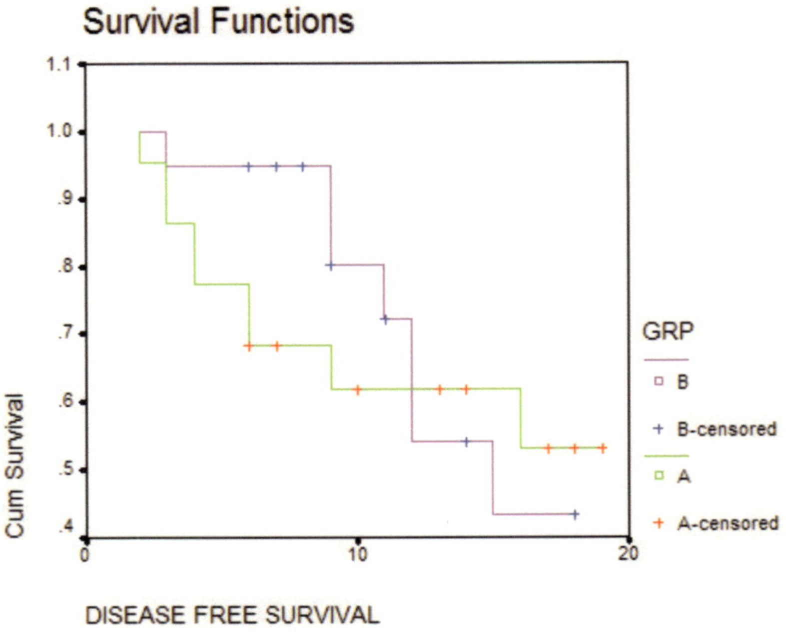

Fig. 24. Patient survival as calculated by Kaplan Meier method

7. References

Robbins KT. Classification of neck dissection: current concepts and future considerations. *Otolaryngol Clin North Am.* Aug 1998;31(4):639-55

Medina JE, Byers RM: Supraomohyoid neck dissection: Rationale, indication and surgical technique.

Head Neck 1989, 11:111-122

Shah JP: Patterns of lymph node metastasis from squamous carcinomas of the upper aerodigestive tract. *Am J Surg* 1990, 160:405-409.

Michael J. Gleeson Scott-Brown's Otorhinolaryngology: Head and Neck Surgery 7Ed , Chapter 199

Medina JE. Neck Dissection. In: Bailey BJ and Johnson JT. *Head & Neck Surgery-Otolaryngology*. 2. 4th ed. Chapter 113: Lippincott Williams & Wilkins; 2006:1585-1609

Ashok R. Shaha Radical Neck Dissection. Operative Techniques in General Surgery, Vol 6, No 2 (June), 2004: pp 72-82

Javier Gavilan et al, Modified Neck dissection. Operative Techniques in General Surgery, Vol 6, No 2 (June),2001: pp 83-94

3

Roles of Therapeutic Selective Neck Dissection in Multidisciplinary Treatment

Muneyuki Masuda, Ken-ichi Kamizono, Hideoki Uryu, Akiko Fujimura and Ryutaro Uchi
Department of Otolaryngology and Head and Neck Surgery, Kyushu Koseinenkin Hospital, 1-8-1 Kishinoura, Nishiku, Kitakyushu , Fukuoka Japan

1. Introduction

In the treatment of head and neck squamous cell carcinoma (HNSCC), management of cervical lymph nodal metastases has a crucial impact on the prognosis of patients. The "radical neck dissection (RND)", which was proposed by Crile (Crile, 1906) in 1906, had long been played a role of standard treatment for neck metastases due to its high curability. However, during the last two to three decades, modified neck dissection (MND), also called as "functional neck dissection", which preserves non-lymphatic structures, has replaced the position of RND, because patients as well as surgeons have become more aware of the significance of the quality of life. In addition, it has become apparent that under current multimodality treatment protocols, MND can achieve improved functional results without compromising oncological outcomes, compared to the conventional RND (Ferlito et al., 2003). Of note, in this study, MND implies the comprehensive (I-V) ND that is generally termed as "modified radical neck dissection (MRND)", unless described otherwise. Moreover, the detailed studies on the patterns of potential neck metastases clearly demonstrated that the laryngeal and pharyngeal cancers seldom metastasize to the level I and V, while the oral cavity cancers to the level IV and V (Lindberg, 1972; Shah, 1990). These data have strongly encouraged the application of selective neck dissection (SND) that spares the dissection of at least one level in the treatment of clinically N0 neck as "elective" SND (ESND). It is now widely accepted that ESND can achieve similar regional control rates compared to comprehensive neck dissection (CND) (i.e., RND or MRND) in this N0 clinical setting with improved functional outcomes as summarized in a comprehensive review (Ferlito et al., 2006). Recent remarkable advancements in chemoradiation have further extended the application of SND to clinically N+ cases as "therapeutic" SND (TSND) instead of therapeutic CND (TCND). Efficacy of TSND performed either as an initial treatment or as a planed ND (PND) in the course of multidisciplinary treatments has been reported by an increasing number of studies (Ambrosch et al., 2001; Byers et al., 1999; Ferlito et al., 2009; Lohuis et al., 2004; Muzaffar, 2003; Patel et al., 2008; Shepard et al., 2010). Moreover, a recent study by Robins et. al., (Robbins et al., 2005) demonstrated that super selective (i.e., only two levels) neck dissection can achieve quite favorable outcomes, when performed as a PND after RADPLAT. In view of these observations, neck dissection (ND) has been recognized as a part of the multidisciplinary treatments composed of surgeries and concurrent chemoradiotherapy (CCR) in our institute. Consequently, we have applied MND as well as less extensive SN in both elective and therapeutic settings to patients with HNSCC, based on relatively simple principals. In this study, we have evaluated the efficacy of our application of ND.

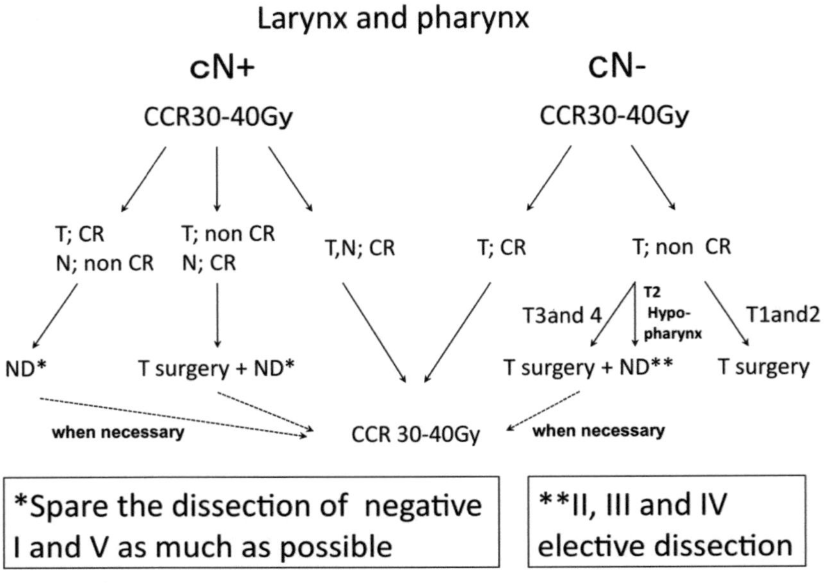

Fig. 1. Algorisms for the treatment of laryngeal and pharyngeal cancers

2. Patients and method

2.1 Eligibility and background of patients

Enrolled patients to this study were primary HNSCC patients who: (1) could have accomplished our protocol-based treatments with curative intent (Figs. 1 and 2), (2) underwent ND during primary treatment course and (3) had been followed more than 12 months. Based on a chart review of HNSCC patients who had been treated at the Department of Otolaryngology, and Head and Neck Surgery, Kyushu Koseinenkin Hospital, from June 2004 to June 2010, 66 subjects were selected. There were 55 male and 11 female. Their ages ranged from 34 to 80 with an average of 62.1. The primary tumors sites were: nasopharynx (n = 3), mesopharynx (n = 16), hypopharynx (n = 14), larynx (n = 11), oral cavity (n = 21), and primary unknown (n = 1). Clinical stage was determined using the 6th UICC TNM classification (2002). T stage was categorized as T1a (n = 1); T1 (n = 5); T2b (n = 1); T2 (n = 21); T3 (n = 20); T4a (n = 14); and T4b (n = 3), N stage as N0 (n = 14); N1 (n = 10); N2 (n = 2); N2a (n = 5); N2b (n = 26); N2c (n = 6); and N3 (n = 2), and clinical stage as I (n = 0); II (4); III (n = 15); Iva (n = 32); and IVb (n = 4). Of note, one primary unknown case was excluded from T and clinical stage classification. Thus, 63.6% (42/66) of patients displayed ≧N2 necks and 78.5% (51/66) of patients were categorized as having stage III-IV advanced HNSCCs. The median follow-up period was 34.1 months ranging from 7 - 85 months.

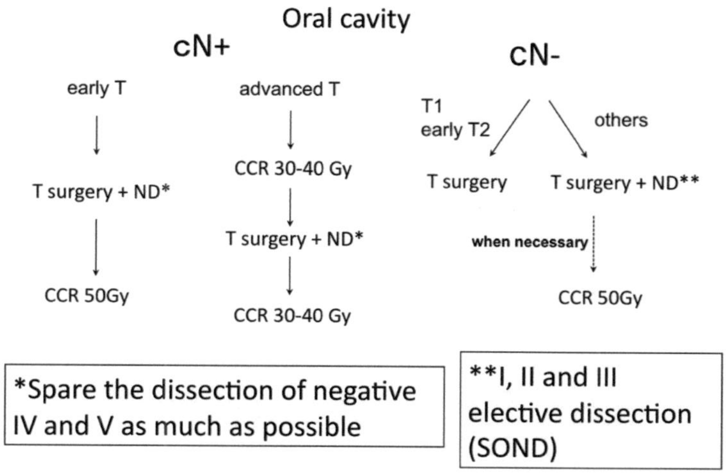

Fig. 2. Algorisms for the treatments of oral cavity carcinomas

2.2 Treatment protocol

All patients, expect for one primary unknown case, were treated with our treatment protocols shown in Figs. 1 and 2.

Briefly, tumors from the pharynx and larynx (Fig.1), and oral tumors with advanced T and N+ (Fig.2) were initially treated with 30-40 Gy of concurrent chemoradiotherapy (CCR) composed of S-1 (80-120mg/day, p.o.), Vitamin A (50.000 IU/day, i.m.) and external beam of irradiation (1.8-2.0 Gy/day), which we have termed "TAR therapy" (Kumamoto et al., 2002; Nakashima et al., 2005). Then further treatments course were determined according to the algorism demonstrated in Figs.1 and 2.

For oral cavity tumors with early T and N+ or any T and N0, surgery was adopted as an initial treatment modality and then additional CCR was administered when necessary. One primary unknown case underwent an initial ND and additional 50 Gy of CCR. In these protocols, ND has been considered as a part of multidisciplinary treatment, and therefore organ preserving ND and both elective and therapeutic SND have been employed as our standard option for neck metastases. Our basic policies for ND are as follows: (1) preserve the spinary accessory verve (XI), internal jugula vein (IJV) and sternocleidmastoid muscle (SCM) (of note, the SCM is sacrificed when primary tumor site is reconstructed with a pectoralis major myocutaneous flap), unless direct invasion of tumors is highly suspected, (2) in N+ cases, the dissection of positive N levels is mandatory, but omit the dissection of respective I and V for laryngeal and pharyngeal cancer and IV and V for oral cavity cancer (Figs. 1 and 2), considering the size, position, number and invasiveness of the positive N located in the adjacent levels, and (3) in N0 cases, we employ ESND: II, III, and IV dissection for laryngeal and pharyngeal cancer, and I, II, and III dissection for oral cavity cancer (i.e., SOND) (Figs. 1 and 2). These protocols are approved by the Hospital Review Board.

2.3 Neck dissection

2.3.1 RND

Fig.3 demonstrates the surgical view of RND for primary unknown bulky nodes and consequent cosmetic and functional results. Deformity of the dissected neck and shoulder-drop are prominent. He has severe difficulty in stretching up of the left arm.

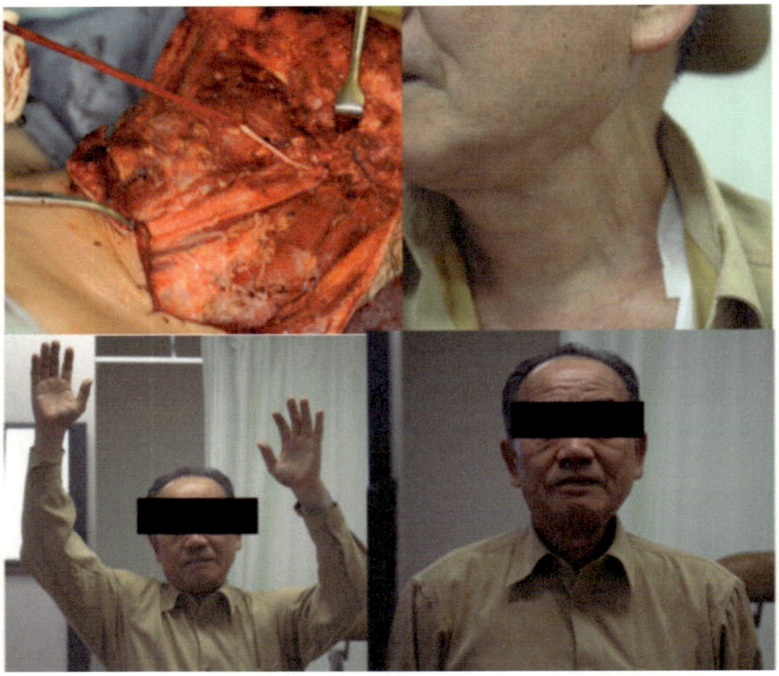

Fig. 3. RND

2.3.2

Fig.4 displays the surgical view of MRND performed during a pull-through glossectomy. The SCM muscle was sacrificed for the reconstruction with a PMMC flap.

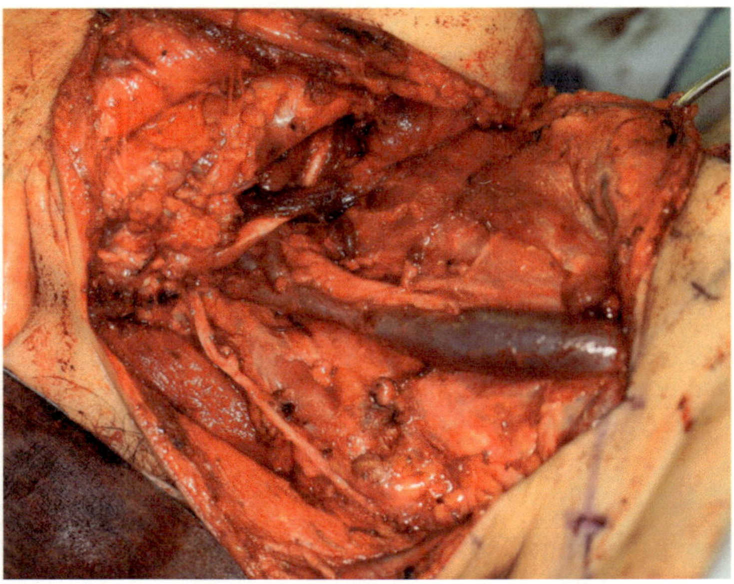

Fig. 4. MRND

2.3.3

Fig.5 displays the surgical view of TSND (II-IV) for mandibular preserving pull-through oropharyngectomy (Masuda et al., 2010). In addition to the XI nerve, SCM and IJV, the facial vein, the external jugular vein, the great auricular and the cervical nerves were preserved.

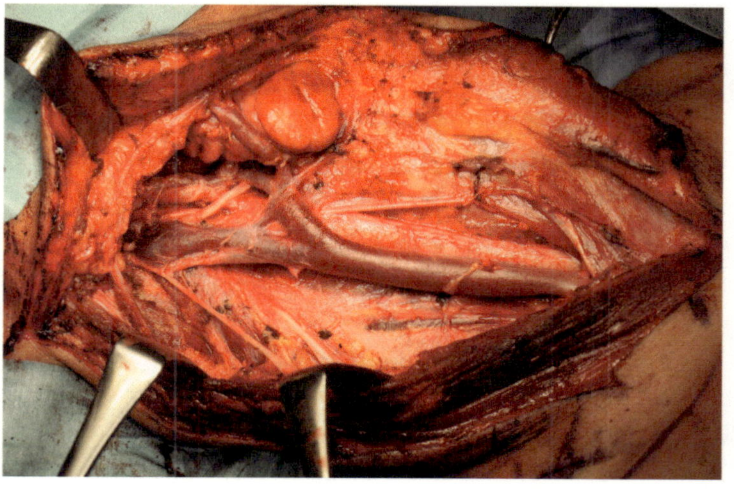

Fig.5. TSND

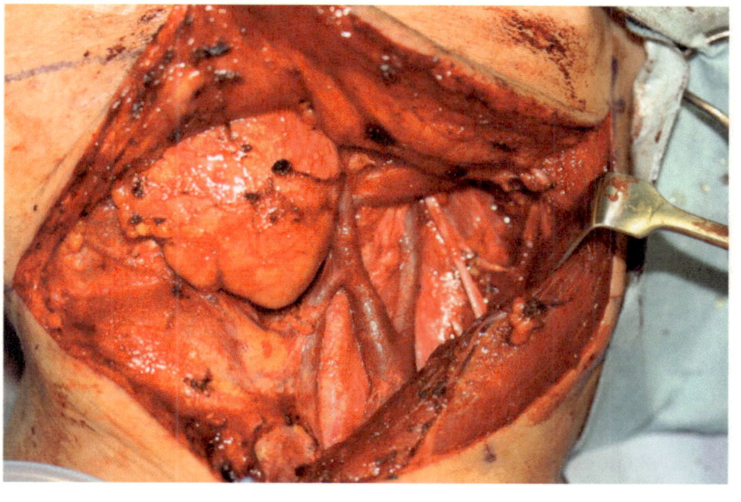

Fig. 6. SOND

2.3.4

Postoperative view of SOND (I-III) performed as an ESND (Fig.6). In this case, the submandibular gland, facial vein, external jugular vein and great auricular nerve were preserved, as well as the XI nerve, SCM and IJV

2.4 Treatment course

Under these protocol-based treatments, 66 patients received 78 NDs. According to the status of nodal metastases and the type of ND they received, 78 necks were divided into 4 groups (Fig.7). Among 15 N0 necks, Group1 (n = 12) underwent ESND, while Group 2 (n = 3) received CND (MRND). For 63 N+ necks, 36 TSNDs were administered to Group 3, while 27 TCNDs (20 MRNDs and 7 RNDs) to Group 4. Except for 3 cases in Group1 and 1 case (pN0) in the Group 3, CCR was administered to 94.9 % (74/78) of cases.

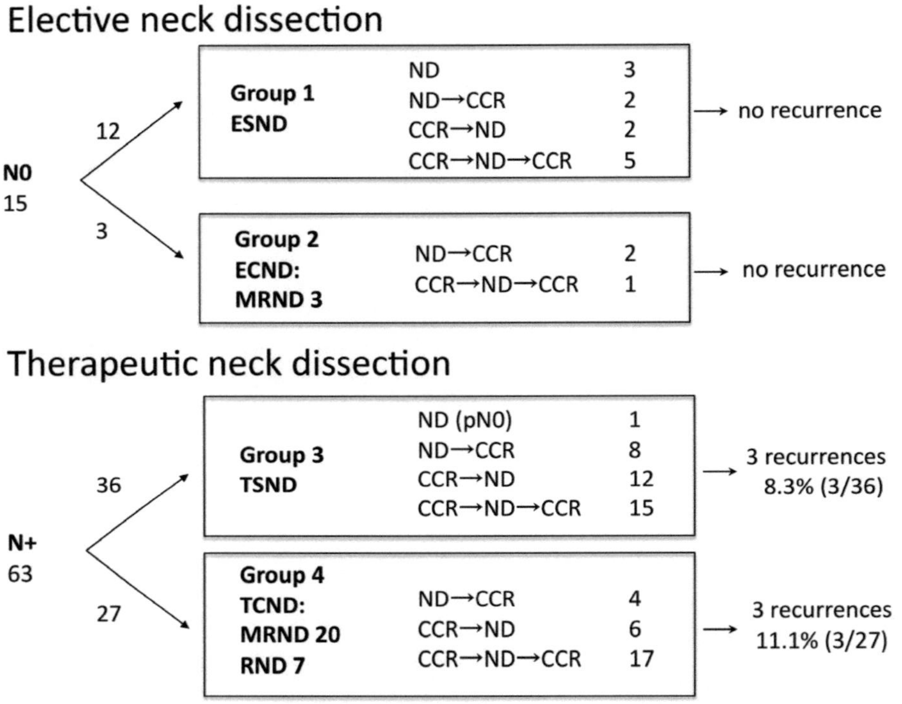

Fig. 7. Grouping of the 78 necks based on the status of nodal metastases and treatment courses

3. Results

3.1 Non-lymphatic structures and level preserved

Conventional RNDs were applied for 7 N+ cases, accounting for only 9% of all NDs. In more than 90% of cases, at least one of the XI nerve, SCM, or IJV was preserved. The detail with respect to organ preservation is shown in Table.1. The XI nerve and SCM were left intact in more than 80% of cases and the SCM in 55.1% of cases. The lowest preservation rate of the SCM among these three organs was due to its sacrifice for reconstruction by a PMMC flap. All the three XI nerve, SCM, and IJV were spared in approximately half (47.4%) cases.

In 21 necks with oral cavity cancer, the dissection of level III, IV and V was omitted at 9.5%, 33.3% and 66.7%, respectively. For 56 necks with laryngeal and pharyngeal cancer the preserving rates of respective I, IV and V were 50.1%, 14.0% and 49.1% (Table.2).

One patient with primary unknown neck metastases (N2b) was treated with RND (Fig. 3).

Preserved organ	Rate of preservation
Spinal accessory nerve	80.1% (63/78)
Sternocleidmastoid m.	55.1% (43/78)
Internal jugular vein	82.0% (64/78)
Two of three	78.2% (61/78)
All three	47.4% (37/78)

Table 1. Organ preservation rates

Tumor Site	Level preserved (%)				
	I	II	III	IV	V
Oral cavity (n = 21)	0	0	9.5	33.3	66.7
Larynx & pharynx (n = 56)	50.1	0	0	14.0	49.1

Table 2. Level preserved

3.2 Distribution of Clinical Stage in SND and CND

In Table 3, the clinical stages of dissected necks were categorized based on the type of neck dissection: SND or CND. A majority of cases in both groups belonged to the advanced stage: 93.5% in SND and 100% in CND. This difference was not statistically significant. A primary unknown case was excluded from this analysis.

Type of ND											
SND						CND					
	NO	N1	N2	N3	total		NO	N1	N2	N3	total
T1	0	0	3	0	3	T1	0	1	1	1	3
T2	3	4	10	0	17	T2	0	1	4	2	7
T3	4	1	8	0	13	T3	3	1	6	0	10
T4	5	3	6	0	14	T4	0	0	10	0	10
total	12	8	27	0	47		3	3	21	3	30

Stage III : 9 (19%) Stage IV : 35 (74.5%)

Stage III : 6 (20%) Stage IV : 24 (80%)

Table 3. Comparison of the clinical stages between SND and CND

3.3 Local control and survival

The 78 dissected necks developed 6 (6.8%) recurrences, which were observed in the cases that underwent therapeutic ND (i.e., Group 3 and Group 4) (Fig.7). The recurrence rate was

8.3%(3/35) in Group 3 with TSND and 11.1 % (3/27) in Group 4 with CND. All 6 recurrences occurred in the dissected levels. Extracapsular spread of dissected nodes was observed in 50% (3/6) of recurrent cases: 1 case in Group 3 and 2 cases in Group 4, and caused the death of the patient. The remaining three recurrences without extracapsular spread, 2 in Group 3 and 1 in Group 4, have been surgically salvaged so far. The cumulative regional control rates, disease specific survival rates and overall survival rates were plotted with the Kaplan-Meier method, comparing the results of SND to those of CND (Fig.8).

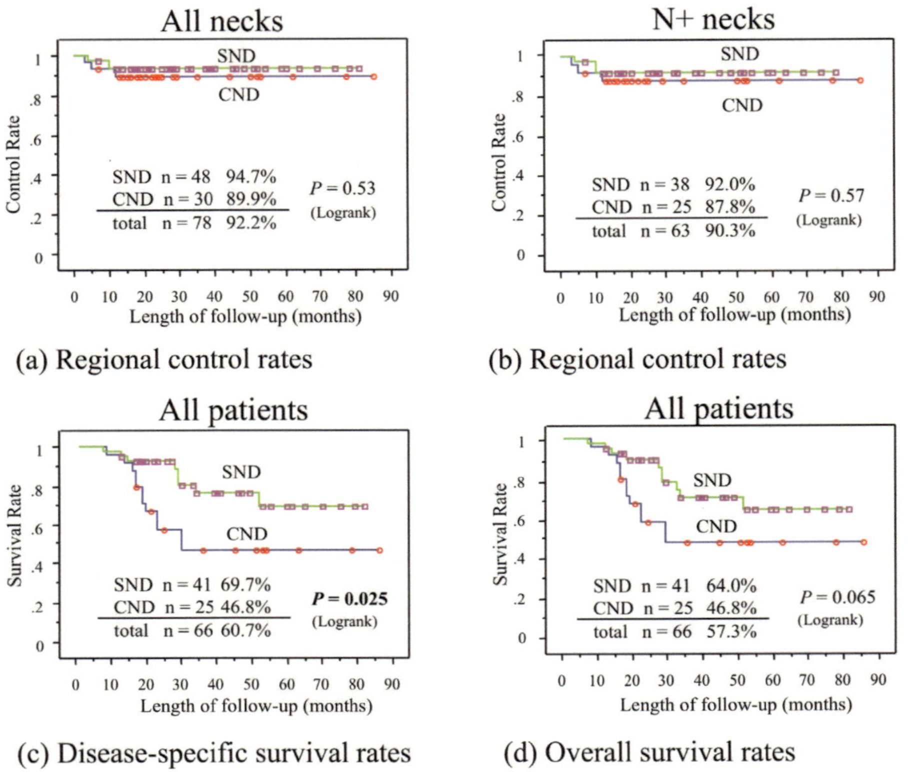

Fig. 8. The Kaplan-Meier plots for regional control and survival rates

In the overall (SND + CND) analysis, quite favorable regional control was obtained in the cohort of all necks (92.2%) (Fig. 8a) as well as in the cohort of N+ necks (90.3%) (Fig.4b). There was a tendency that the regional control rate of SND was higher than those of CND, thus SND yielded 94.7% in all necks and 89.9% in N+ necks, while CND 89.9% in all necks and 87.8% in N+ necks (Figs.8a and 8b). However, these differences were not statistically significant in the comparison studies by the Logrank test. The cumulative and over all disease specific survival rates were 60.7% and 57.3%, respectively (Figs. 8c and 8d). In the disease specific analyses, the SND group displayed significantly (P = 0.025) better prognosis (69.7%) than the CND group (46.8%)(Fig.8c). This tendency was also observed in the overall survival curves, but the difference between SND (64%) and CND (46.8%), was not statistically significant (P = 0.065) (Fig.8d).

3.4 Causes of deaths

In the present study, 22 deaths were observed. Twenty patients were died with causes related to the primary cancer: distant metastases, (n = 10), metastases to the Rouviere node (n = 2), primary tumor recurrence (n = 4), nodal metastases in the un-dissected neck (n = 2), and nodal metastases in the dissected neck (n = 3). The remaining two deaths were unrelated to the primary tumor: accident and pancreatic cancer. Consequently, regional failures in both dissected and un-dissected necks accounted for only 22.7 % (5/22) of deaths. Moreover, only 3 regional failures in the dissected necks were responsible for the deaths. More detail about regional failures of the dissected necks is described above.

4. Discussion

4.1 SND for N0 necks

The efficacy of SND for N0 necks as an elective ND has been confirmed by a solid body of evidence (Ferlito et al., 2003; Ferlito et al., 2006). Thus, it is not surprising that in the present study there were no recurrences in Group 1 undergoing ESND as well as in Group2 undergoing ECND (Fig.3). This high control rate might also be attributable to the fact that as many as 75 % (9/12) of necks in Group 1 received CCR. Thus, application of ESND for N0 necks, especially when they are treated with multidisciplinary treatment, seems to be adequate for selected patients.

4.2 TSND in multidiciplinary treatment

In accordance with the trend of multidisciplinary treatment, TSND has gained a wider acceptance in the treatment of HNSCCs. In general, TSND has been applied under two different lines of treatment regimens: (1) as an initial surgery followed by radiotherapy (Ambrosch et al., 2001; Byers et al., 1999; Lohuis et al., 2004; Muzaffar, 2003; Patel et al., 2008; Shepard et al., 2010), or (2) as a planned ND following CCR (Ferlito et al., 2009). In the former regimen, the indication of adjuvant radiotherapy was not uniform and in some studies it was mandatory but in others it was given to selected patients with risks including extracapusular spread, multiple pathological nodes and advanced T stage. However, irrespective of the application pattern of adjuvant radiotherapy, the regional recurrence rates of SND were 3-13% and more importantly theses figures were equivocal to or lower than those of CND in the studies that compared these two cohorts. The latter regimen apparently reflects the recent paradigm shift of the treatment for advanced HNSCCs. Thus, the current mainstay is induction CCR - in particular, dose-intensified - followed by a planned ND (PND). It was clearly demonstrated in a recent comprehensive review (Ferlito et al., 2009) that by means of SND or super SND, equivalent and safer results can be obtained compared to more extensive ND, although the indication of PND to cases that displayed complete response after CCR is now raising a hot debate.

In view of these two lines of regimens, our treatments protocols seem to be unique and lie at the intermediate between them. Thus, except for the early stage oral cancers, for which surgery has been reported to be more efficient than external irradiation, CCR is administered first. Then, at 30-40 Gy of CCR, we screen responders who can proceed to organ preservation arm; a screening method we have termed "chemoradioselection". Since 1972, we have used this method for approximately 40 years for the treatments of HNSCC, achieving high organ preservation and survival rates especially in laryngeal cancer (Kumamoto et al., 2002). Similar concept of "chemoselection" has been recently proposed by the group of University of Michigan (Urba et al., 2006; Worden et al., 2008; Worden et al., 2009). They demonstrated that those who display favorable responses to induction chemotherapy tend to be cured by additional chemoradiotherapy without surgical intervention, facilitating organ preservation.

Considering the above mentioned trend for less extensive ND in the context of our treatment concept, we have applied organ preserving MND and SND in both elective and therapeutic clinical settings for the treatment of HNSCC. The aim of this study was to evaluate the efficacy of our application of ND, in particular, that of TSND. In both clinical settings, quite favorable regional control rates (84.7-94.7%) were obtained (Figs. 4a and 4b). These figures are similar to or better than those reported in the studies mentioned above. Thus, it is apparent that high organ preservation rates in the present study (Table 1) do not compromise regional control. Furthermore, it is also demonstrated that our indication of ND determined in the algorism-based protocols (Fig. 1 and 2) is quite acceptable. In conclusion, when employed under a definite principal, TSND is a reliable alternative to MRND and RND in multidisciplinary treatment.

In addition to the high regional control rates, patients in the present study displayed relatively favorable disease-specific (60.7%) and overall (57.3%) survival (Figs. 4c and 4d), although 77 % of patients had advanced stage. This is, at least in part, due to the high regional control rates observed in both SND and CND cohort, thus only 5 patients died with regional failure. However, in both disease-specific and overall survival analyses, the CND cohort displayed apparently poor prognosis, reflecting the aggressiveness of the initial tumor status of this population that led to deaths unrelated to the regional failure (e.g., distant metastases, the Rouviere nodal metastases and primary tumor recurrences). This finding might imply the limit of our treatment protocol. However, considering that the survival rates of this study is favorable even compared to those obtained by the recent dose-intensified types of treatment protocols summarized in a recent review (Ferlito et al., 2009), it seems to be quite challenging to develop a practical countermeasure to improve the prognosis of this population with highly aggressive tumors.

5. Conclusions

Organ preserving SND in both elective and therapeutic clinical settings is a quite reliable alternative to more aggressive ND (i.e., RND and MRND), when properly applied in multidisciplinary treatment.

6. Acknowledgement

This study was supported in part by fund from Grants-in-Aid for Scientific Research (C): 21592195 to Muneyuki Masuda

7. References

Ambrosch P. et al (2001). Efficacy of selective neck dissection: a review of 503 cases of elective and therapeutic treatment of the neck in squamous cell carcinoma of the upper aerodigestive tract. *Otolaryngol Head Neck Surg* 124: 180-7, 0194-5998

Byers R.M. et al (1999). Selective neck dissections for squamous carcinoma of the upper aerodigestive tract: patterns of regional failure. *Head Neck* 21: 499-505, 1043-3074

Crile G. (1906). Excision of cancer of the head and neck. With special reference to the plan of dissection based on one hundred and thirty-two operation. *JAMA* 47: 1780-86

Ferlito A. et al (2009). Planned neck dissection for patients with complete response to chemoradiotherapy: a concept approaching obsolescence. *Head Neck* 32: 253-61, 1097-0347

Ferlito A. et al (2003). Changing concepts in the surgical management of the cervical node metastasis. *Oral Oncol* 39: 429-35, 1368-8375

Ferlito A. et al (2006). Elective and therapeutic selective neck dissection. *Oral Oncol* 42: 14-25, 1368-8375

Kumamoto Y. et al (2002). "FAR" chemoradiotherapy improves laryngeal preservation rates in patients with T2N0 glottic carcinoma. *Head Neck* 24: 637-42, 1043-3074

Lindberg R. (1972). Distribution of cervical lymph node metastases from squamous cell carcinoma of the upper respiratory and digestive tracts. *Cancer* 29: 1446-9, 0008-543X

Lohuis P.J. et al (2004). Effectiveness of therapeutic (N1, N2) selective neck dissection (levels II to V) in patients with laryngeal and hypopharyngeal squamous cell carcinoma. *Am J Surg* 187: 295-9, 0002-9610

Masuda M. et al (2010). Mandible preserving pull-through oropharyngectomy for advanced oropharyngeal cancer: A pilot study. *Auris Nasus Larynx* 38: 392-7, 1879-1476

Muzaffar K. (2003). Therapeutic selective neck dissection: a 25-year review. *Laryngoscope* 113: 1460-5, 0023-852X

Nakashima T. et al (2005). [Phase I study of concurrent radiotherapy with TS-1 and vitamin A (TAR Therapy) for head and neck cancer]. *Gan To Kagaku Ryoho* 32: 803-7, 0385-0684

Patel R.S. et al (2008). Effectiveness of selective neck dissection in the treatment of the clinically positive neck. *Head Neck* 30: 1231-6, 1097-0347

Robbins K.T. et al (2005). Effectiveness of superselective and selective neck dissection for advanced nodal metastases after chemoradiation. *Arch Otolaryngol Head Neck Surg* 131: 965-9, 0886-4470

Shah J.P. (1990). Patterns of cervical lymph node metastasis from squamous carcinomas of the upper aerodigestive tract. *Am J Surg* 160: 405-9, 0002-9610

Shepard P.M. et al (2010). Therapeutic selective neck dissection outcomes. *Otolaryngol Head Neck Surg* 142: 741-6, 1097-6817

Urba S. et al (2006). Single-cycle induction chemotherapy selects patients with advanced laryngeal cancer for combined chemoradiation: a new treatment paradigm. *J Clin Oncol* 24: 593-8, 1527-7755

Worden F.P. et al (2008). Chemoselection as a strategy for organ preservation in advanced oropharynx cancer: response and survival positively associated with HPV16 copy number. *J Clin Oncol* 26: 3138-46, 1527-7755

Worden F.P. et al (2009). Chemoselection as a strategy for organ preservation in patients with T4 laryngeal squamous cell carcinoma with cartilage invasion. *Laryngoscope* 119: 1510-7, 1531-4995

4

Complications of Neck Dissection

Nader Saki and Soheila Nikakhlagh
Cancer Research Center of Ahvaz Jundishapur University of Medical Science, Iran

1. Introduction

Head & neck cancer is the major problem due to its associated morbidity and mortality. It is the sixth most common cancers and the eighth cause of cancer mortality in the world(1). The most important prognostic factor in the management of head and neck cancer is the presence of cervical lymph node metastasis. Neck dissection has been a well-established procedure for diagnosing (staging) and treating head and neck cancer for almost a century(2). This procedure is used to eradicate metastases to the regional lymph nodes of the neck. Since Crile introduced radical neck dissection at the beginning of the 20th century, a few changes have been proposed by Hays Martin in 1951 and Suárez which aimed for a more conservative approach to preserve vital anatomical structures in the neck without compromising the completeness of lymph node removal. The transition from radical to selective neck dissection has resulted in fewer complications and lower morbidity, at the same time preserving surgical efficacy and compliance with oncologic principles.(4)

Depending on the location and extent of the tumor, the type of neck dissection performed may be radical, modified, selective and extended and either unilateral or bilateral. Complications of neck dissection affect every surgeon regardless of experience and technical skill. In addition to the various medical complications that may occur after any surgical procedure in head & neck region, a number of surgical complications may be related to the neck dissection. Complications of neck dissection are divided into three major categories: wound complications, Nerve complications, Vascular complications. Co-morbidities such as cardiac, respiratory and hepatic disease are common place in patients undergoing neck dissections in either an elective or therapeutic sense. Additional immunosuppression caused by conditions such as diabetes or relative malnutrition should be optimised since they predispose to complications including as wound infection. (5)

2. Prevention of complications

A careful history begins any thorough surgical evaluation. The surgeon should inquire about prior surgery and tumor therapy. Previous neck surgery may have an impact on incision design. Careful study of the lesion to be excised is of great importance. Its precise location, size, firmness, and mobility with respect to surrounding structures should be noted(6). Prior radiation therapy also slows healing, thus heightening the risk of postoperative complication. Patients should be encouraged to cease smoking as long before surgery as possible. Smoking exacerbates pulmonary dysfunction and may impair vascular perfusion, resulting in flap loss. The importance of communication between the anaesthetic

and surgical teams cannot be over emphasised. There are theoretical advantages to using low-molecular weight as opposed to standard low dose heparin in the prophylaxis of deep vein thrombosis and pulmonary emboli since it lessens bleeding complications, has a prolonged duration of action and is less likely to induce thrombocytopaenia.(2,7)
Intraoperative events, such as hemorrhage, loss of a venous suture resulting in gas embolism, chylous leakage due to thoracic duct injury, and arrhythmia because of carotid bulb manipulation, are habitually promptly managed; these events may, however, be disastrous for the patient. Careful dissection and ligature of vessels are extremely important to avoid intra-and postoperative hemorrhage. (8)

3. Wound complications

Although preparation of a surgical site prevents wound contamination by removing transient pathological bacteria and decreasing resident flora counts, good surgical technique with minimal tissue damage still has a role to play. Removal of large amounts of beard hair may increase the rate of infection unless carried out immediately prior to surgery. A variety of approaches exist for the approach to neck dissections that usually simply rely on surgeon preference, e.g. martin double-Y incision, apron access(7,9).
The incidence of wound infection after surgery of the neck without entry into the aerodigestive tract should be very low. Prophylactic antibiotics may be continued during the first 24 to 72 postoperative hours. Wound infection is a contributing factor to dehiscence and flap skin loss. Others include poor nutrition, prior radiation therapy, poor incision and flap design, and continued smoking during the perioperative period. Skin Flaps should be elevated in the sub-platysmal plane in order to maximise their blood supply unless local disease dictates otherwise. Flap elevation superficial to the platysma adds to the prolems of skin loss(3,8).(fig1)
Wound infection may manifest as a cellulitis with erythema, warmth, or induration of the cervical skin flaps, abscess formation from an infected seroma or hematoma, or fistula (12). Once a wound infection is detected, action must be taken to minimize sequelae.Wound Complications after neck dissection are associated with increased patient morbidity and hospitalization. Other complications are also possible such as: Undesired Scarring, Flattened Appearance and Pain.

4. Nerve complications

4.1 Sensory branches of the cervical roots

Sensory branches of the cervical roots provide sensation to skin of the neck and shoulder. As the skin flaps are elevated in subplatysmal plane, several branches of the cervical plexus are immediately encountered overlying the SCM. Sacrifice of these branches will results in a sensory deficit that extends from pinna to the chest wall below the clavicle. Most of this sensory deficit will spontaneously resolve postoperatively over a period of months. Branches of the cervical plexus can also form neuromas, which present as firm, painful masses in the lateral neck that are exquisitely tender to palpation(9).

4.2 Greater auricular nerve

The greater auricular nerve serves as an excellent landmark for the proper plane for elevation of the skin flap, because it lies lateral to the SCM. The nerve should be kept down

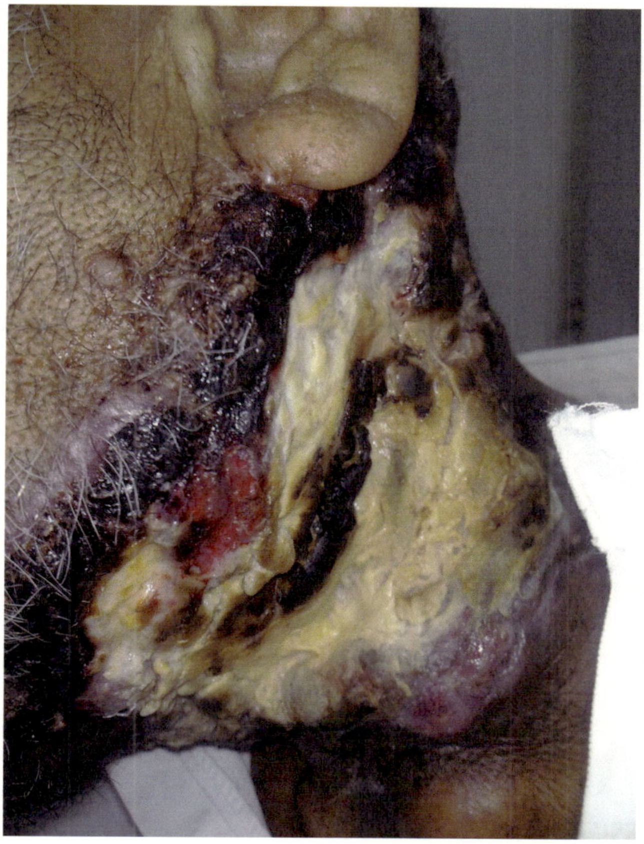

Fig. 1. Wound infection and necrosis

on the SCM during flap elevation, and the decision of whether to preserve it can be made later. Sacrifice of this nerve during neck dissection leads to a sensory deficit of the auricle that usually diminishes with time. Neuroma of divided greater auricular nerve can occur(10).

4.3 Lingual nerve

The lingual nerve is primarily a branch of the mandibular division of the trigeminal nerve(cranial nerve V) that carries general sensation from the anterior two thirds of the tongue. It also receives the chorda tympani nerve from the facial nerve, which carries taste from the same region of the tongue. Level I neck dissection incorporating submandibular gland excision puts this nerve at risk for injury. Clinically, injury results in loss of taste from ipsilateral anterior two third of the tongue and hypoesthesia or paresthesia of the hemitongue with resultant difficulty with speech and deglutition(4).

4.4 Facial nerve

During standard neck dissection usually the cervical and marginal mandibular branches of the facial nerve are encountered. The Cervical branch of facial nerve innervates the platysma muscle. Sacrifice of the cervical branch does not uaually produce clinically significant deficits.

The marginal mandibular branch of the facial nerve is typically single branch and its position with respect to the body of the mandible is highly variable. Injury to this nerve causes an obvious cosmetic deformity with asymmetry of the motion of the corner of the mouth. The marginal mandibular branch can be preserved by ligation and superior retraction of the facial vein. The branch is thus rolled up with the skin flap and kept away from further surgical dissection(3).

4.5 Spinal accessory nerve

The Spinal accessory nerve consists entirely of motor fibers to the SCM and Trapezius muscle. Prevention of injury of the nerve is achieved by proper identification of the Spinal accessory nerve using standard landmark and meticulous handling of the nerve once identified. Sacrifice of or damage to the Spinal accessory nerve (cranial nerve XI) is a major contributing factor to complaints related to the shoulder. Pain and weakness of the shoulder are among the most common postoperative complications of neck dissection(11).

4.6 Vagus nerve

Whether the surgeon plans to sacrifice or preserve the internal jugular vein, it is necessary to first identify all of the structures in the carotid sheath. Inadvertent injury to the vagus nerve may occur during the process of ligation the internal jugular vein in the inferior neck or at the skull base. High vagus nerve injuries result in significant dysphonia from ipsilateral vocal cord paralysis and dysphagia with pooling of secretions from pharyngeal paralysis and loss of sensation in the larynx. A breathy voice , an inefficient cough, and a subjective sense of dyspnea result. The loss of more distal vagal innervations has little clinical effect(4).

4.7 Hypoglossal nerve

Hypoglossal nerve injury is a rare complication of neck dissection. The nerve is susceptible to injury during dissection of level I,II, near the greater cornu of hyoid bone and adjacent to the carotid artery. Hypoglossal nerve injury result in ipsilateral tongue weakness, deviation of the tongue to the affected side and difficulty with speech and swallowing(5).

4.8 Phrenic nerve

The phrenic nerve arises from C3,C4 and C5 and it courses between the anterior scalene muscle and its overlying fascia. As elevation of the contents of the posterior triangle proceeds from the trapezius toward the carotid sheath, the cervical plexus contributions to the phrenic nerve or to a loop of the phrenic nerve itself may be injured. phrenic nerve paralysis is considered a rare complication of neck dissection and leads to ipsilateral hemidiaphragm elevation with or without mediastinal shift on chest radiograph, and it may contribute to postoperative pulmonary complications. Preservation of the fascial layer over the nerve and anterior scalene muscle is the primary method for prevention of injury. Fluoroscopic examination postoperatively confirms the diagnosis of phrenic nerve injury(6).

4.9 Sympathetic nerve

The fusiform cervical sympathetic gangion consists of two to four ganglia running parallel and deep to the carotid sheath. There is rarely any reason to enter this area during tumor removal in neck dissection, but, injury can occur during retraction of the carotid sheath to clear tumor or adjacent lymph nodes and may be temporary, related to traction or permanent due to transaction. The neurologic deficit caused by injured to the cervical sympathetic nerves depends on the site of injured. A classic Horner syndrome consists of the following ipsilateral conditions: Miosis, Ptosis, Anhydrosis , Transient blush and nasal congestion. No Horner syndrome will results from an injured below the stellate gangion located behind the vertebral artery in the root of the neck(8,11).

4.10 Brachial plexus

Lateral to the phrenic nerve beneath the fascial floor of the posterior triangle is the brachial plexus, which is wedged between the sclanenus muscles. This structure , like the phrenic nerve, is deep to the deep cervical fascia, and it should be easily preserved when gentle blunt dissection of the fat overlying the fascia is performed. Any fat that does not come away from the floor of the posterior triangle with gentle blunt dissection must be cautiously examined to be certain that there is no nerve running within. If a nerve is present, the surgeon must decide whether to dissect it free of the surrounding fat or to leave the fat at the floor of the dissection(8).

5. Vascular complicatioms

5.1 Hematoma

Hematoma occurs in approximately 1% of the neck dissections. Failure to recognize and properly treat a hematoma results in increased wound complications. Prevention consists of preoperative avoidance of anticoagulants and antiplatelet agents and meticulous intraoperative hemostasis. Careful dissection and meticulous hemostasis during surgery are extremely important to avoid intra-and postoperative hemorrhage. Hematomas are avoided by careful hemostasis, application of pressure dressing and continuous suction drainage. Most introperative complications may be prevented by means of careful surgical technique, coupled with a thorough understanding anatomy of head & neck(8).

5.2 Internal jugular vein complications

It is important to clear the upper jugular nodes thoroughly, because they are common sites for tumor recurrence. The internal jugular (IJ) has several large tributaries that enter it anterosuperiorly. If it is to be spared, care must be taken to ligate these branches well away from the wall off the preserved vein. Narrowing of the vein probably contributes to the postoperative thrombosis and occlusion that are reported to occur in 15% of preserved jugular vein. Thrombosis of the internal jugular (IJ) vein is an underdiagnosed condition that may occur as a complication of head and neck infections, surgery, central venous access, local malignancy, polycythemia, hyperhomocysteinemia, neck massage, and intravenous drug abuse. It is also reported to occur spontaneously. IJ thrombosis itself can have serious potentially life-threatening complications that include systemic sepsis, chylothorax, papilledema, airway edema, and pulmonary embolism. The diagnosis often is very challenging and requires, first and foremost, a high degree of clinical suspicion. If the Internal jugular vein is to be ligated during neck dissection, it should first be thoroughly exposed, with the position of the vagus and hypoglossal nerves being noted(7).

5.3 Carotid artery complications

Complications involving the common carotid artery are the most feared sequelae of neck surgery. Acute postoperative carotid artery rupture, or "blow out" occurs in 3% to 4% of radical neck dissection and associated with a mortality rate of 50%. Factors associated with carotid artery hemorrhage include wound breakdown, necrosis, and infection, pharyngocutaneous fistula, prior radiation therapy, tumor involvement of the arterial wall. Tumor invasion of the carotid artery is a relatively uncommon event of advanced aggressive disease or revision surgery for a recurrent neck mass(4).when wound dehiscence results in the exposure of the carotid artery,it is more ominous, and its management more critical.(fig2)

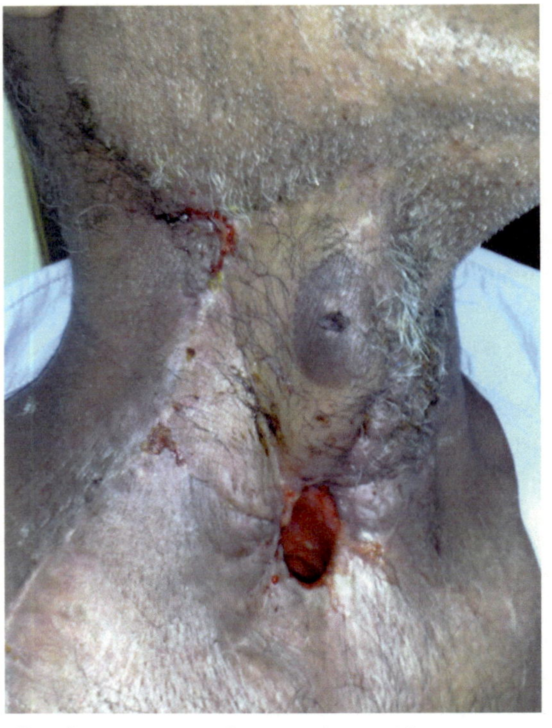

Fig. 2. Pectoralis major flap for coverage of exposed carotid artery

5.4 Chyle fistula

The thoracic duct arises from the cisternal chyli at the level of the second lumbar vertebra and rises into the neck between the aorta and the azygos vein. In the thorax it crosses to the left and after passing behind the aortic arch and left subclavian artery it lies on the anterior scalene muscles and phrenic nerve. The duct terminates most commonly in the left IJV although less commonly it may enter the left subclavian, left external jugular, left brachiocepalic (innominate) vein or right IJV. Up to 50% of patients exhibit more than one termination of the duct. The right lymphatic duct drain terminates at the junction of the right subclavian vein and IJV. The key to treatment of a chyle fistula is prevention which demands knowledge of the relevant anatomy. Whereas intra-operative identification can be aided by placing the patient in the Trendelenburg position or adopting a forced Valsalva manoeuvre, post-operative leaks are usually identified when feeding is commenced. Multiple approaches to the treatment of an established leak have emerged including nutritional, surgical and pharmalogical therapy. Although there are strong feelings amongst clinicians about the use of bowel rest, parental nutrition or low fat enteral formulae for the treatment of established chyle leaks, definitive evidence supporting one therapy over another does not exist (4).

6. Conclusion

Surgery of the neck requires a high level of expertise and familiarity with the complex anatomy of the region. Complications in neck surgery may occur despite the best efforts to prevent them. Proper preoperative planning, early recognition of perioperative complications, and prompt, effective management can minimize the impact of complications that may occur.

7. References

[1] Kazi, RA. "The Life and Times of George Washington Crile: An Outstanding Surgeon." The Internet Journal of Otorhinolarygology. 2003. Vol 2, No 2.

[2] Shaha, A. 2007. "Editorial: Complications of Neck Dissection for Thyroid Cancer." Annals of Surgical Oncology. Accessed: August 19, 2010. Available at: *http://www.ncbi.nlm.nih.gov/pmc/articles/PMC2244697/.*

[3] Ferlito, A et al. Neck Dissection: past, present and future? J. Laryngol Otol. 2005 (1) 1-6.

[4] Smoke A, Delegge MH: Chyle leaks: consensus on management? *Nutr Clin Pract* 2008, 23(5):529-32. PubMed Abstract | Publisher Full Text

[5] Walker FD, Cooke LD: Antimicrobial prophylaxis in otorhinolaryngology/head and neck surgery. *Clin Otolaryngol* 2007, 32(3):204-7. PubMed Abstract | Publisher Full Text

[6] Lauchlan DT, McCaul JA, McCarron T: Neck dissection and the clinical appearance of post-operative shoulder disability: the post-operative role of physiotherapy. *Eur J Cancer Care (Engl)* 2008, 17(6):542-8. PubMed Abstract | Publisher Full Text

[7] Prim MP, De Diego JI, Verdaguer JM, Sastre N, Rabanl I:Neurologic complications following neck dissection .*Eur Arch Otorhinolaryngol* 2006, 263(5):473-6. PubMed Abstract | Publisher Full Text

[8] Tatla T, Kanagalingam J, Majithia A, Clarke PM: Upper neck spinal accessory nerve identification during neck dissection. *J Laryngol Otol* 2005, 119(11):906-8. PubMed Abstract | Publisher Full Text

[9] Weiss KL, Wax MK, Haydon RC 3rd, Kaufman HH, Hurst MK: Intracranial pressure changes during bilateral radical neck dissections. *Head Neck* 1993, 15(6):546-52. PubMed Abstract | Publisher Full Text

[10] Brown DH, Mulholland S, Yoo JH, Gullane PJ, Irish JC, Neligan P, Keller A: Internal jugular vein thrombosis following modified neck dissection: implications for head and neck flap reconstruction. *Head Neck* 1998, 20(2):169-74. PubMed Abstract | Publisher Full Text

[11] Prim MP,De Diego JI,Verdaguer JM. Neurological complications following functional neck dissection. Eur Arch Otorhinolaryngol.2006;263(5):473-476.

[12] Nader Saki, Soheila Nikakhlagh , Maryam Kazemi. Pharyngocutaneous Fistula after Laryngectomy: Incidence, Predisposing Factors, and Outcome. Arch Iranian Med 2008; 11 (3): 314 - 317

Part 3

Advances and Modification of Neck Dissection

5

Lateral Cervical Flap a Good Access for Radical Neck Dissection

Raja Kummoona
Professor Emeritus of Maxillofacial Surgery Acting Chairman of Maxillofacial Surgery Iraqi Board for Medical Specializations, Baghdad Iraq

1. Introduction

An important and vital area of the head &neck entail the coverage of defects throughout the head and neck area. These defects usually covered by flaps, during the last 6 decades since the introduction of tube pedicle flap till the early sixty of the last century (Macgregor 1960) advocated his temporal fascial flap for coverage of intra oral defect after radical cancer surgey, this flap was a great advancement of radical surgery in the oro facial region. Advocation of flaps represent an artistic and fully acceptable of the nose, cheek, tongue, floor of the mouth, chin and neck.1,2,3

We know that blood supply was important for survival of flaps and we have to pay attention to the distinct arterial and venous supply of any flap.Axialflaps such as musculocutanous flaps,fascio cutanous flaps and micro vascular free flaps were introduced in the decades of 1970,these flaps were rapidly used to greater number with clinical application in head and neck area and the concept of <delay> of flaps has been a banded and no more accepted as a method for reconstruction of the oro facial region.

Flaps in general can be designed to be of an adequate dimensions and knowledge of its vascular supply and to be assured of a consistut satisfactory and acceptable result. Many flaps been advocated that differ not only in their design, type of flaps based on theblood supply is concerned. A number of soft tissue flaps have been used to reconstruct the oro facial region after ablative surgery , also random flaps been used successfully such as delto pectoral and cervico pectoral flaps but with limitation on use of these flaps in old people due to atherosclerosis. The aim is to repair the defect created by resection of tumor or a defect of post traumatic missile injuries of the face to restore function and provide an acceptable cosmetic feature. 3, 4,6,8,9

2. Indication of Lateral Cervical Flap

1. Design of the flap and its elevation superiorly making a good access to resection of the mandible, supra omohyoid neck dissection, modified radical neck dissection and classical radical neck dissection, since other techniques forming a band of scar extended along the neck at the site of radical neck dissection

2. It's an excellent flap for reconstruction of the tongue, floor of the mouth, alveolus and cheek after radical cancer surgery of oro facial region
3. It is a superior flap for reconstruction of the chin and sub mental area in cases with post traumatic missile injuries of the lower third of the face.
4. Platysma muscle flap is an excellent flap for reconstruction of atrophied masseter muscle in cases of mild first arch dysplasia syndrome and also used to invest the chondro-osseous graft for reconstruction of the TMJ and condyle

3. Anatomy of the flap

The lateral cervical flap (LCV) comprises skin, fascia and platysma muscle. Success in utilizing the LCV depends on through understanding on its anatomy and vascular supply. The clavicle forms the lower boundary of the lateral neck, the mandible, the superior border along with the mastoid process of the temporal bone and superior nuchal line of the occipital bone. It extends posterior to the anterior border of trapizeus muscle and is divided obliquely by the sternocliedomastoid muscle into the anterior and posterior triangles of the neck.

The major structures of the neck are surrounded by the investing layer of deep fascia which encloses the sternocliedomastoid and trapizeus muscles forms the roof of posterior triangle. The deep investing fascia is pierced by the cutanous branches of the cervical plexus, the external jugular vein and small cutanous arteries. The superficial cervical fascia is not a separate layer but a zone of loss connective tissue between the dermis and deep fascia and is continuous with both. This fascia covers the platysma muscle and contains a considerable amount of fat tissue. In many places the deep part of the superficial fascia contains muscle fibers. These muscle fibers are striated and are similar to the muscles of facial expression.Immediatly below and deep to the superficial fascia is a layer of deep fascia.

The platysma muscle represent the lower part of expression muscles; it originates from the deep fascia that covers the upper part of pectorals major and deltoid muscles it passes upward into the neck as thin muscular layer or sheet embedded in the deepest layer of superficial fascia and reaches to the lower border of the mandible. The posterior fibers enter the face and blend with the muscles of the lower lip and lip commisure.In this region the inferior labial artery and terminal branches to the cheek supply the muscle fibers of platysma.Below the chin the anterior fibers interlace and blend with the muscle fibers of the opposite side. The motor nerve is the cervical branches of facial nerve and the sensory supply comes from the cutanous nerves of the overlying skin.

Superiorly the LCV is supplied by the superficial branches of occipital and posterior auricular arteries. The major arterial supply of the platysma muscles comes from sub mental artery a branch from facial or faciolingual arteries. Additional blood supply comes to platysma muscle from inferior labial artery and from other terminal branches of external carotid arteries. The venous drainage of this area via the external jugular vein laterally and via anterior jugular vein medially.

The occipital artery originates from the posterior aspect of the external carotid artery deep to the lower border of the posterior belly of digastrics muscle and runs to the occipital groove of the temporal bone. In most cases it pierces the fascia between the attachment of sternocliedomastoid and trapizus muscles or passes through muscle fibers of sternocliedomastoid muscle to sub cutanous tissue in its terminal superficial branches. It

supplies the muscles of the neck and back of the head and the arteries of scalp anastomose freely with each other and with the opposite side.
Posterior auricular artery is a small branch of the external carotid artery, arises at the level of superior margin of the digastrics muscle or sharing a common trunk with the occipital artery. It ascend between the auricular cartilage and the mastoid process and divide into auricular and occipital branches and both arteries anastomos freely.1,2

4. Operative technique and design of flap

The LCV which includes skin, fascia and muscle can safely be elevated as superiorly based flap with rich blood supply coming from superficial branch of occipital artries, the posterior auricular artery and sub mental branch of facial artery.Demage to the sub mental branch during elevation of the flap has little effect on viability of the flap.
Two parallel vertical incisions are made one start just below the mastoid region and the other begins below the lower border of the mandible and 2cm anterior to the masseter muscle, both vertical incisions extend down to the clavicle, the free part of the flap which include skin, fascia and muscle is elevated and passed through a tunnel under the angle of the mandible into the mouth. The flap can be used for reconstruction of the tongue after hemi glasso ctomy or alveolus after radical resection of the mandible or reconstruction the floor of the mouth or reconstruction of the cheek after radical cancer surgery of the cheek. The flap can be used for reconstruction of sub mental region and chin following post traumatic missile injuries of the orofacial region there is no need fo tunnel to be used.1,2 ,Fig 1

5. Experimental studies

Experimental studies done by the author in 8 growing rabbits 3 months of age and approximately of 1.6Kg body weight. They were divided into 2 groups; 4 each group and these further subdivided into 2 left and 2 rights sided. Each group of 4 subjected to different operation. The first group had hemiglossactomy done on 2 animals each side and in the second group of 4, apiece of skin excised from sub mental area of about 6cm diameter excised on 2 sides of the animals. Surgical procedures via full thickness LCF incisions on each side of the rabbit neck were done. Flap was immediately transferred for reconstruction of the tongue on 4 rabbits,2 each side and also the flap was used for reconstruction of sub mental area immediately after creation of defect in the second group of 4 rabbits 2 left and 2 right.1
This procedure was done under ketamine hydrochloride sedation(Vitalar) 50mg/kg of body weight with infiltration of the tongue and sub mental area by local anesthesia (Lignocaiene hydrochloride 2% with adrenaline1/80000).All animals returned to their cages and were allowed to take their normal usual diet.
The result of this experiment, all animals showed no restriction of mouth opening nor difficulties in mastication and by the end of experiment after 3 months, all animals showed good health and the tongue examined after reconstruction byLCF showed excellent healing with smooth tongue due to desquamation of the skin flap to meet the requirement of functional demand of the masticatory process for the hard food of the rabbits with no evidence of hair growing in the tongue after reconstruction of the defect by LCF.while in the second group the LCV were used for reconstruction of sub mental area the LCF showed growing hair in the area that been reconstructed by LCF.This study proved high viability of LCF.Fig 2

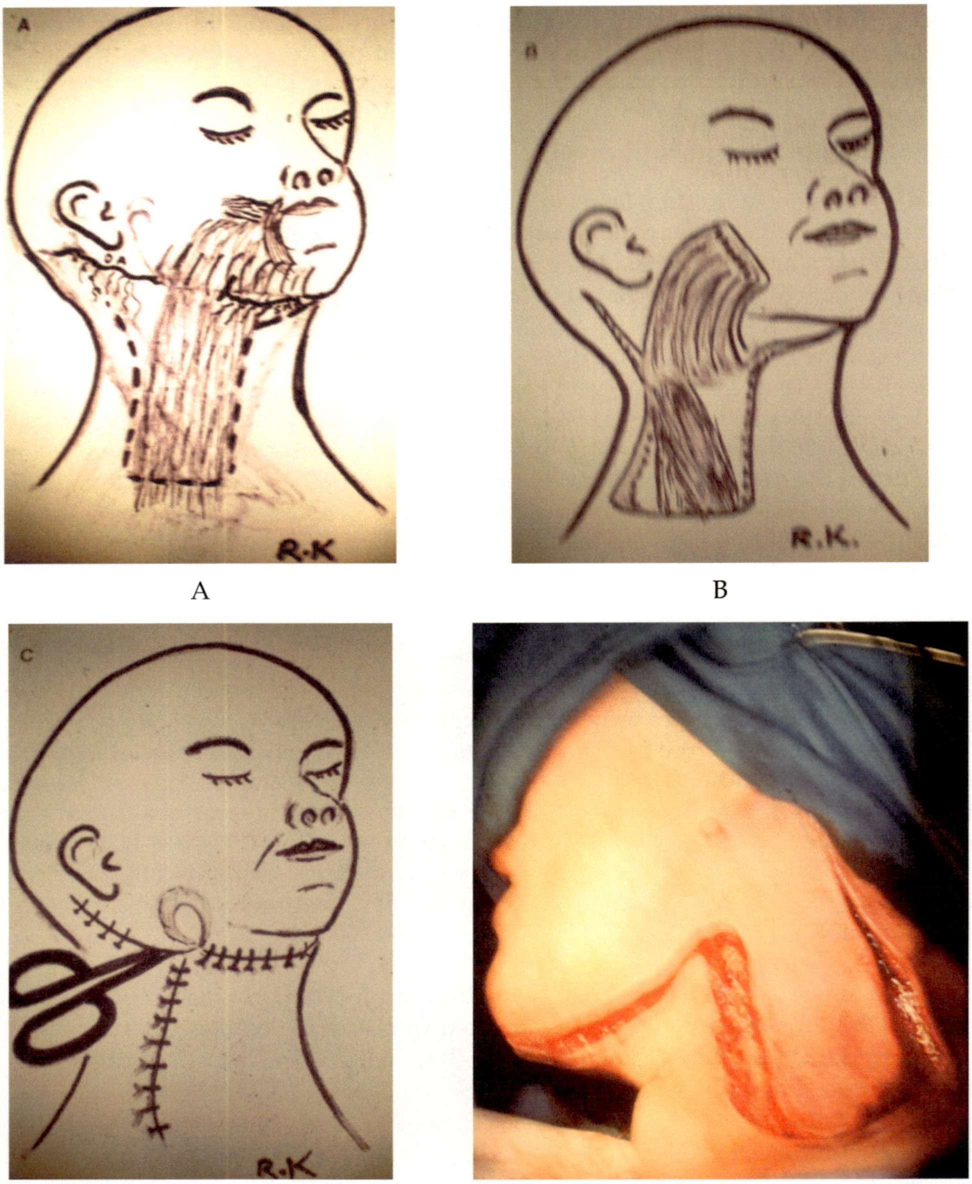

Fig. 1. Diagrams showing, A-Design of lateral cervical flap, B-Elevation of LCF, C-Insertion of LCF, D-Incision of LCF

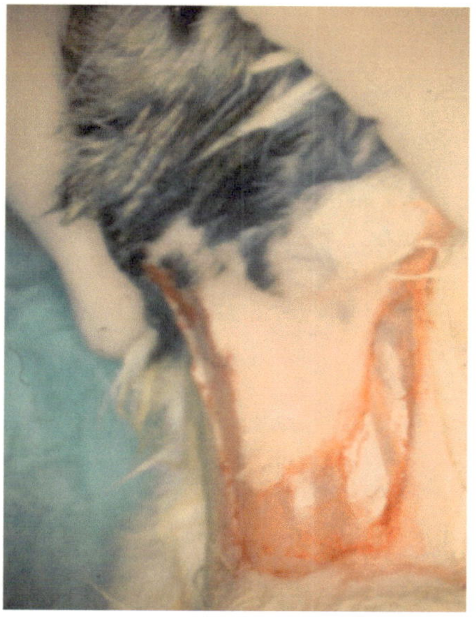

A

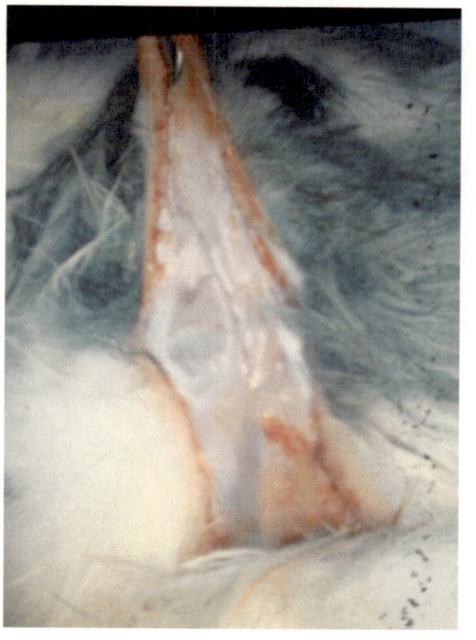

B

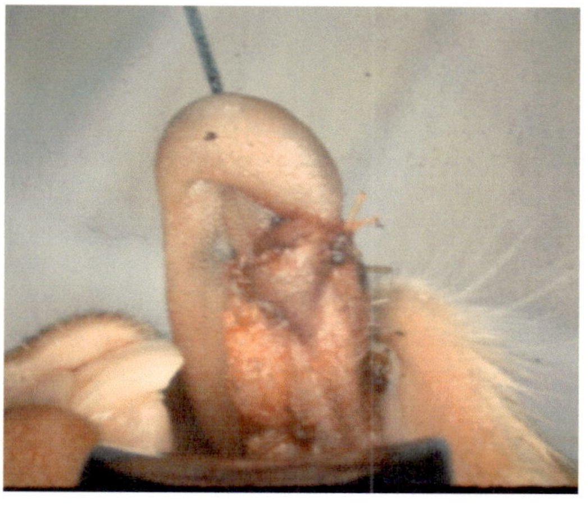

C

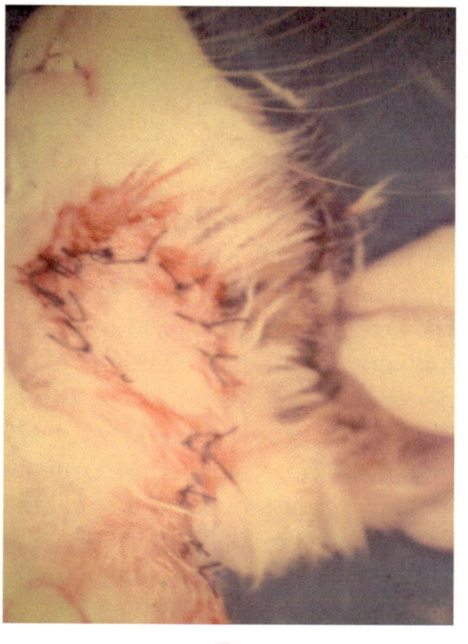

D

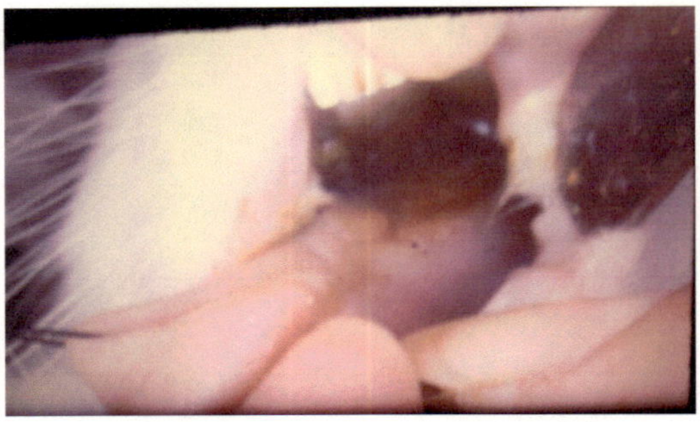

E

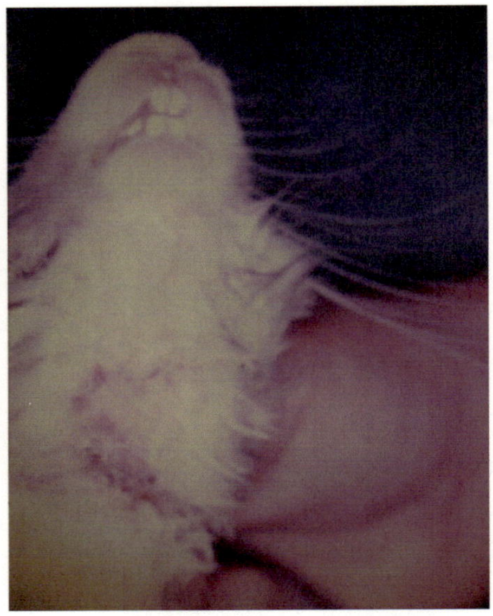

F

Fig. 2. Experimental studies. A-Design of incision of LCF in rabbit, B-Elevation of LCF in the neck of rabbit, C-LCF used for reconstruction of the tongue rabbit after hemiglossactomy, D-LCF used for reconstruction of sub mental region in a rabbit, E-Post operative after 3 months showing excellent healing of the tongue of a rabbit with desquamations of the flap, F-Post operative photograph showing good healing of the flap in sub mental area with growing hair in the reconstructed area

6. Clinical result

This study including 75 patients and these patients were follow-up for 3-6 years,37 were males and 38 females with a median age of 46 years (range 3-81years).They were treated in the Maxillofacial unite, Hospital of Specialized Surgery, Medical City, Baghdad during a period of 6 years, sixty-one patients with oral squamous cell carcinoma including 25 cases with well differentiated squamous cell carcinoma,24 cases with moderately differentiated squamous cell carcinoma and 12 cases of poorly differentiated squamous cell carcinoma. These cases were studied for the proliferative activity of squamous cell carcinoma by AgNOR staining and electron microscopy, also in 24 patients with oral carcinoma an expression of Bcl2 proto-oncogene in tumor tissue and the oral mucosa of the same patients were used as control. In 23 cases of oral carcinoma, the LCFwas used an excess for supraomo hyoid neck dissection and 10 cases of posttraumatic missile injuries of orofacial region and 4 cases platysma muscle flap were used for reconstruction of atrophied masseter muscle.

7. Study of proliferative activity of oral carcinoma

Study of the proliferative activity of squamous cell carcinoma by using an electron microscope(EM) which is an important tool used in cancer research and ultra structural pathology of most malignant tumors. This EM can be used alone or with other technique like nuclear organizer regions (AgNOR) in oral carcinoma.AgNOR are a set of proteins associated with DNA segments(loop called rDNA) that transcribe to ribosome RNA.These proteins are defined as markers of <active> ribosomal genes responsible for protein synthesis.5

The nuclear organizer regions are segment of ribosomal DNA located on the short arm of the five areocentric chromosome 2,11,13 in the nucleoli of cells, previous studies neither of AgNOR as indicators of precise proliferation status have resulted in ambiguity.

The silver nuclear organizer region impregnation technique can be used for studding the number, size and shape neither of NOR in a fast and simple way not only in fresh frozen sections but also in formalin fixed paraffin embedded material. The amounts of silver deposit in the cells reflect the amount of NORS involved in protein synthesis related to proliferative activity of the cell.

This study evaluated the role of AgNOR for assessment the proliferative activity and the cytopathological changes in poorly differentiated oral squamous cell carcinoma by EM.

8. Study of anti apoptotic gene of oral carcinoma by using Bcl2 oncogene

The cellular compartment in tissue is maintained by a finally orchestrated balance between input (Proliferation) and output (Differentiation and Apoptosis) processes. Abnormalities in these mechanisims lead to cancer.10

Bcl2 was first described in follicular lymphoma that beret 14:18(q32,q21) translocation. This structural chromosomal aberration leads to over production of Bcl2 messenger RNA and protein Bcl2 is localized at outer mitochondrial and nuclear membrane as well as in endoplasmic reticulum.Bcl2 proto-oncogene belong to family of apoptosis. The action of Bcl2 oncoprotien is to inhibit apoptosis and is expressed by many tumors including carcinoma of the breast, cervix and head and neck.10

9. Application of LCF

In 23 cases of oral carcinoma the LCV was used as an excess for radical supra omohyoid neck dissection,10 cases of post traumatic missile injuries and 4 cases of platysma muscle was used for reconstruction of atrophied masseter muscles in mild hemi facial microsomia

10. Result

The study result of proliferative activity of the cells by using AgNOR staining and EM.All sections were stained with AgNOR stain for examination of the proliferative activity of the squamous cell carcinoma and biopsies also were performed for another 6 cases ,3 with normal oral mucosa and 3 cases with normal striated muscle from the oral cavity of patients with oral squamous cell carcinoma to serve as control.

Statically studies of AgNOR scores were classified into 3 scores. The P value of score I of analysis variance(ANOVA) test was 0.0001, score II (ANOVA)test was 0.0001 and score III (ANOVA)test was 0.06.Both score 1 and score 2 were highly significant and score 3 was significant.5

11. Electron microscopy study

EM showed tumor cells with irregular shape and size, with remarkable divisions of nuclei and chromatin clumps emarginated toward nuclear membrane. Some cases showed chromatin condensed in one pole of nucleus, few mitochondria with dilated cristea and abundant rough endoplasmic reticulum were observed and few apoptotic changes were noticed.7

These finding showed a high proliferation in poorly differentiated squamous cell carcinoma and the amount of AgNOR in this type of tumor was a prognostic factor and represent unfavorable prognostic features in squamous cell carcinoma.

The study result of anti apoptotic gene of oral carcinoma by using Bcl2 oncogene, we found the expression of Bcl2 proto oncogene in tumor tissue derived from 24 patients with malignant oral carcinoma and normal mucosa from same patients served as control and showed a cytoplasmic pattern of Bcl2 immunoreactivity in basal cell layer. Fourteen of 24 cases represent (58.3%) of oral carcinoma and 4 adenocystic carcinoma expressed positive Bcl2 oncogene.

Well differentiated squamous cell carcinoma (G1) showed absence of immunoreactivity and with no statistically significant correlation could be demonstrated between Bcl2 immunoreactivity and the age and sex of the patients or tumor size and lymph node metastasis. We did find a direct correlation betweenBcl2 immunoreactivity in moderately differentiated squamous cell carcinoma (G2) tumor and poorly differentiated tumor (G3) and was statistically significant ($P< 0.05$).Patients with absence or low (scores 0 or 1), Bcl2 immunoreactive tumor manifestated poorer overall survival rate in comparison with patients with moderate or high (scores 2 and3) Bcl2 expression but the differences was not statistically significant.

Tumors showed 3 different expression of Bcl2 (weak, moderate and strong positive) compared to mucosa of same patient effected by these tumors.,10

No correlation was found between the histopathology of the tumors, mucosal expression and degree of Bcl2 expression. We do propose from these finding the over expression of Bcl2 proto-oncogene act as strong antiopototic mechanisms in both squamous cell carcinoma and adenocystic carcinoma and act as an important molecular event on oral carcinoma to make this tumor resistant to radiotherapy and chemotherapy.10

12. Reconstruction by LCF divided into 4 techniques

12.1 The use of LCF as an access for radical neck dissection and resection of intra oral tumors without using the LCF for reconstruction

In this technique raising the LCF as routine for management of intra oral cancer and the flap acting as stand by for reconstruction, but in some cases reconstruction can be achieved by local flap such as tongue flap, cheek flap or nasolabial flap. Elevation of LCF was required for supra hyoid neck dissection.1,2,3,4

12.2 The use of LCV for reconstruction of the oral cavity after radical cancer surgery

The LCV was used in 23 cases of oral carcinoma. Six cases with squamous cell carcinoma involving the lower alveolar bone with extension to the floor of the mouth, these cases were treated by radical resection of the tumor and floor of the mouth and supra hyoid neck dissection, before any surgical procedure s an ultra sonography been used for detection of any deposit in the cervical lymph nodes in operable cases ,eight cases with carcinoma of the tongue was treated by hemiglossoctomy with supra hyoid neck dissection, 6 cases with extensive squamous cell carcinoma of the cheek were treated by radical excision of the cheek and radical resection of the alveolus of the mandible with supra hyoid neck dissection,4 cases were involving the floor of the mouth and treated by wide radical excision of the floor with supra hyoid neck dissection. All cancer cases were treated by radical surgery and supra omo hyoid neck dissection with adjuvant chemotherapeutic regimens (5-Flourauracil 10 mg/m2+ bleomycien 10 U/m2+carboplatien 400mg/m2) of 3 courses and fallowed by DXT and follow up of these cases was between 3-8 years.1,2,3,4,Fig 3,4,5

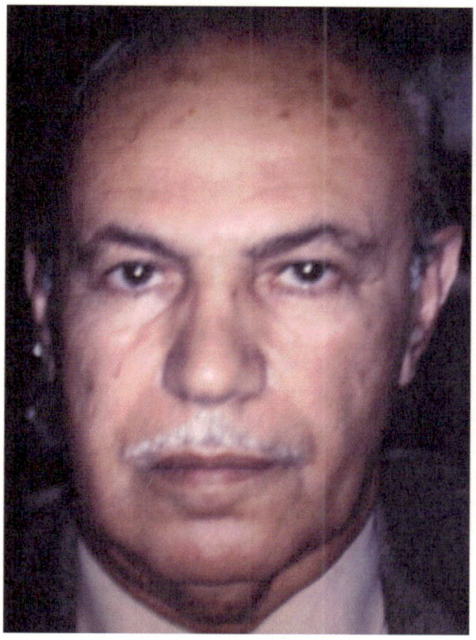

A

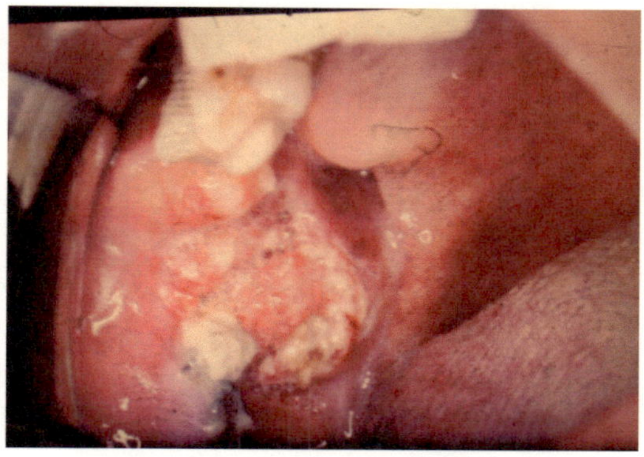

B

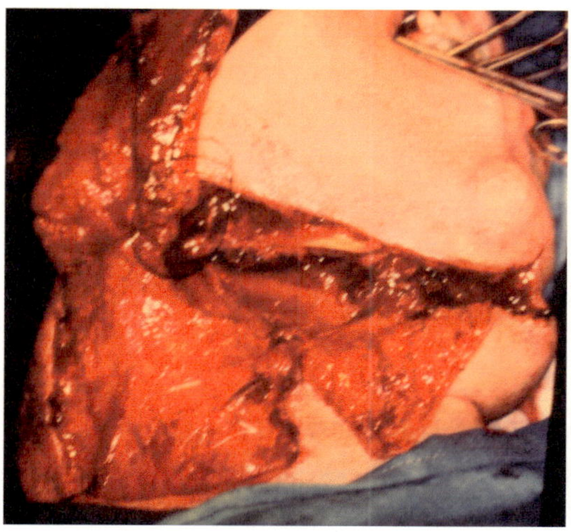

C

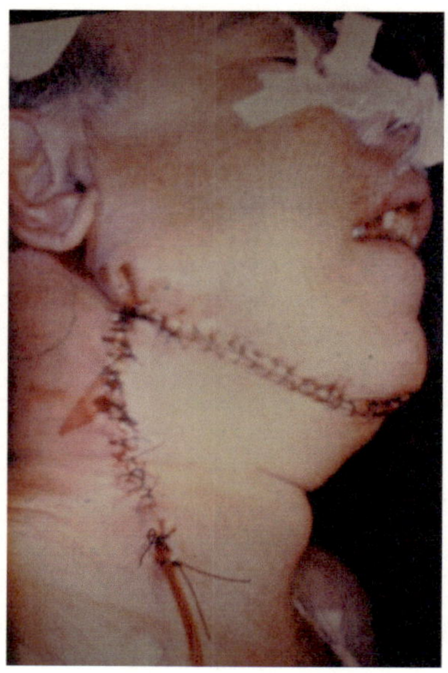

D

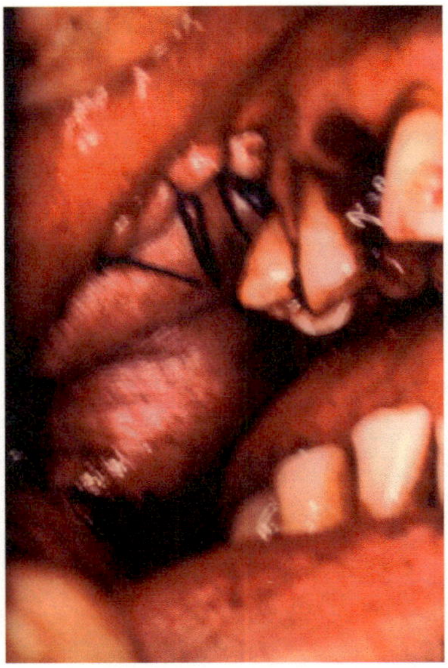

E

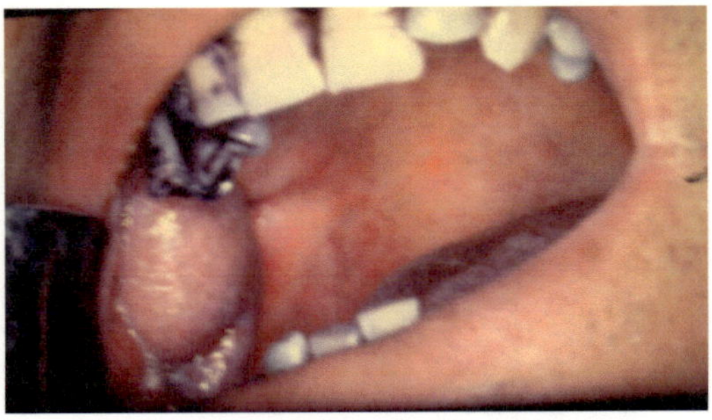

F

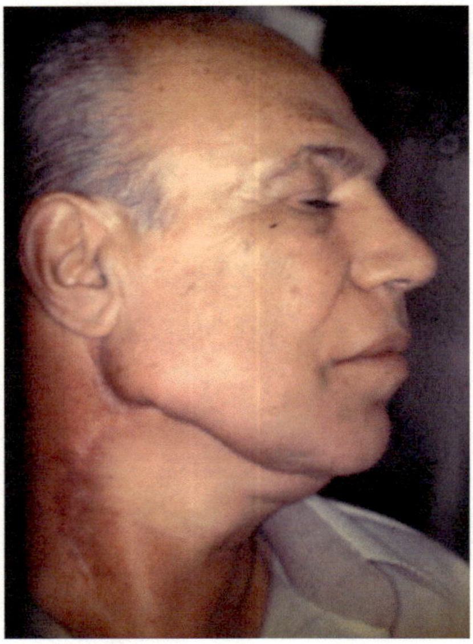

G

Fig. 3. Reconstruction of the cheek by LCF. A-Man of 60 years with ca of the right cheek, B-Extensive squamous cell carcinoma of the right cheek, C-LCF flap elevated after supra omohyoid neck dissection and radical excision of cheek tumor, D-Closure of the neck after LCF been used for reconstruction of the cheek, E-LCF used for reconstruction of the cheek, F-One year after reconstruction of the cheek by LCF, G-Excellent healing of the neck and without showing any vertical band of scar as seen by other technique

Flaps in these cases had an excellent results, in total of 27 cases were diagnosed at stage I,10 cases at stage II,12 at stage III and 12 at stage IV.Twelve patients survived with tumor size of T1 and T2 and the histopathological diagnosis was well differentiated squamous cell carcinoma with no nodal metastasis so far. Most of the patients were lost to follow-up due to instability of the country.

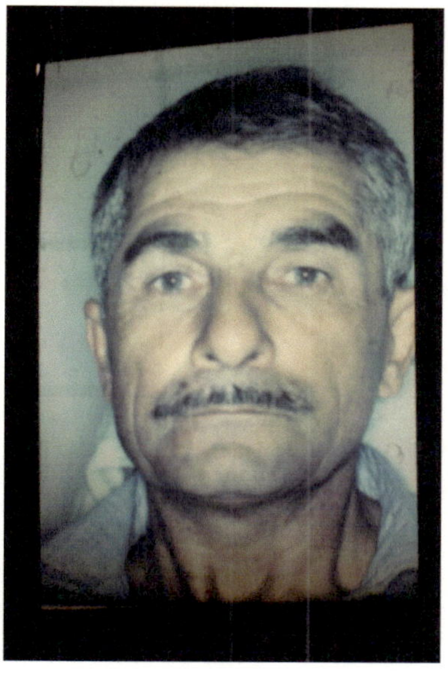

A

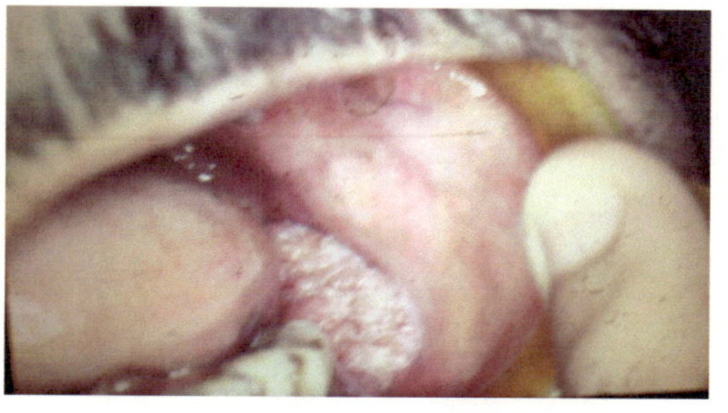

B

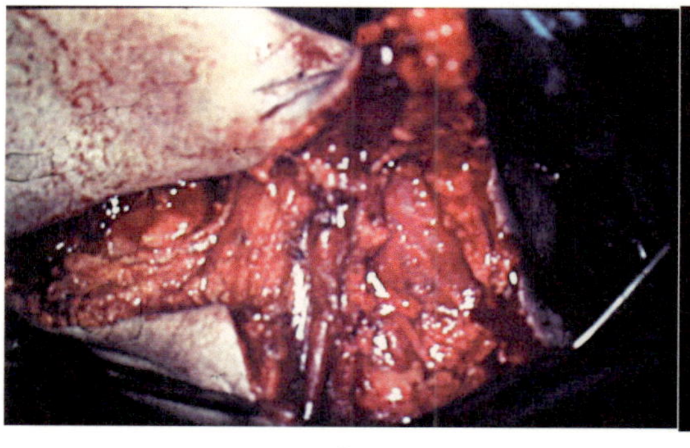

C

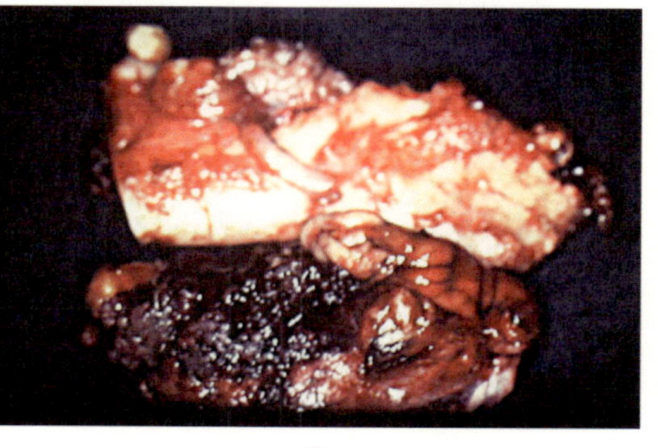

D

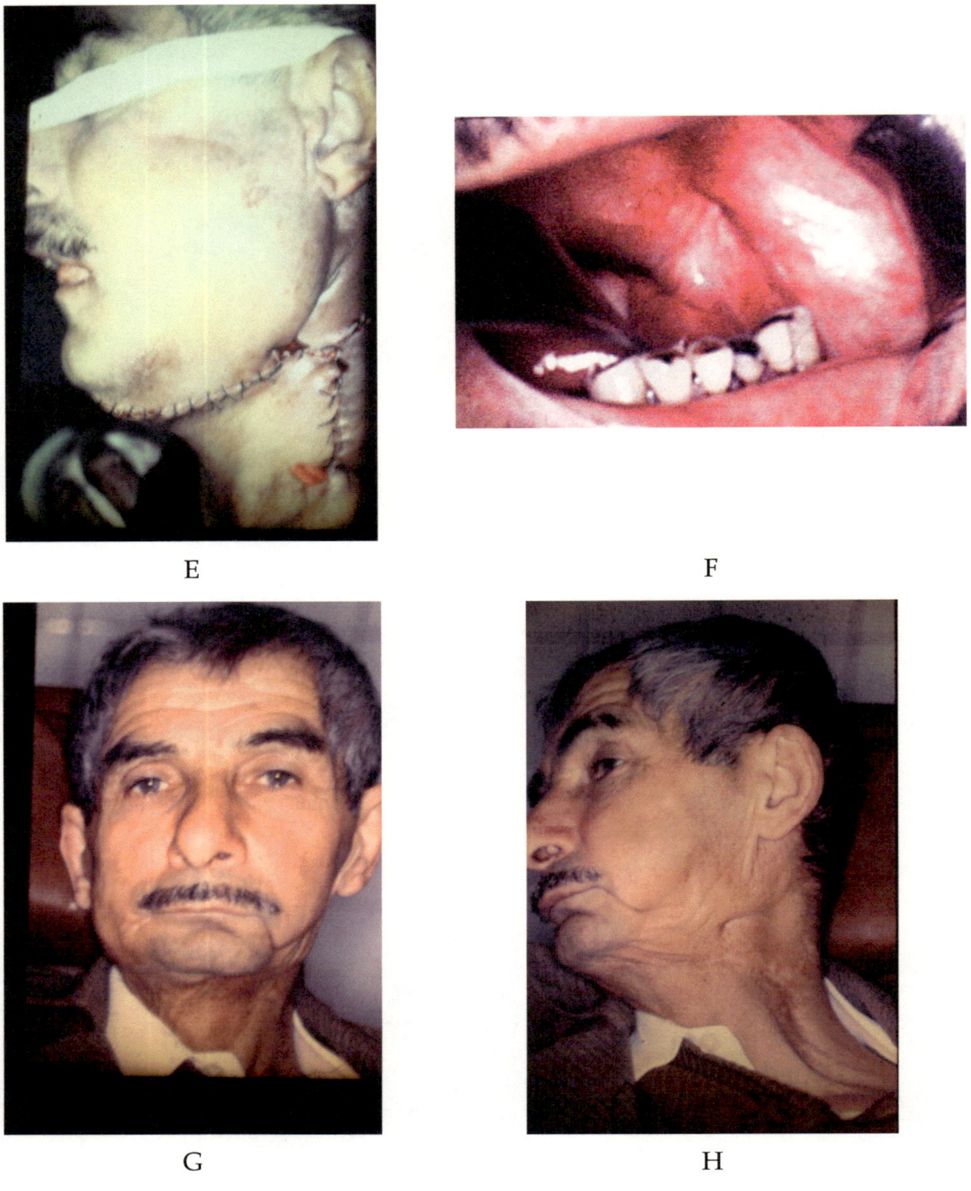

Fig. 4. Reconstruction of the alveolus of the mandible. A-A smoker Man of 60 years with Ca alveolus, B-Extensive squamous cell carcinoma of the alveolus, C-LCF elevated and the anatomy of the neck after supra omohyoid neck dissection and radical resection of the tumor of the mandible, D-Radical resection of the mandible and supra hyoid neck dissection content as showed in the specimen, E-Closure of the neck after LCF been used for reconstruction of the alveolus intra oraly, F-Excellent healing of intra oral defect and alveolus of the mandible after 5 years, G-Post operative photograph after 5 years, H-Lateral side of the neck after LCF used with no vertical band of scars or recurrence masses of lymph nodes

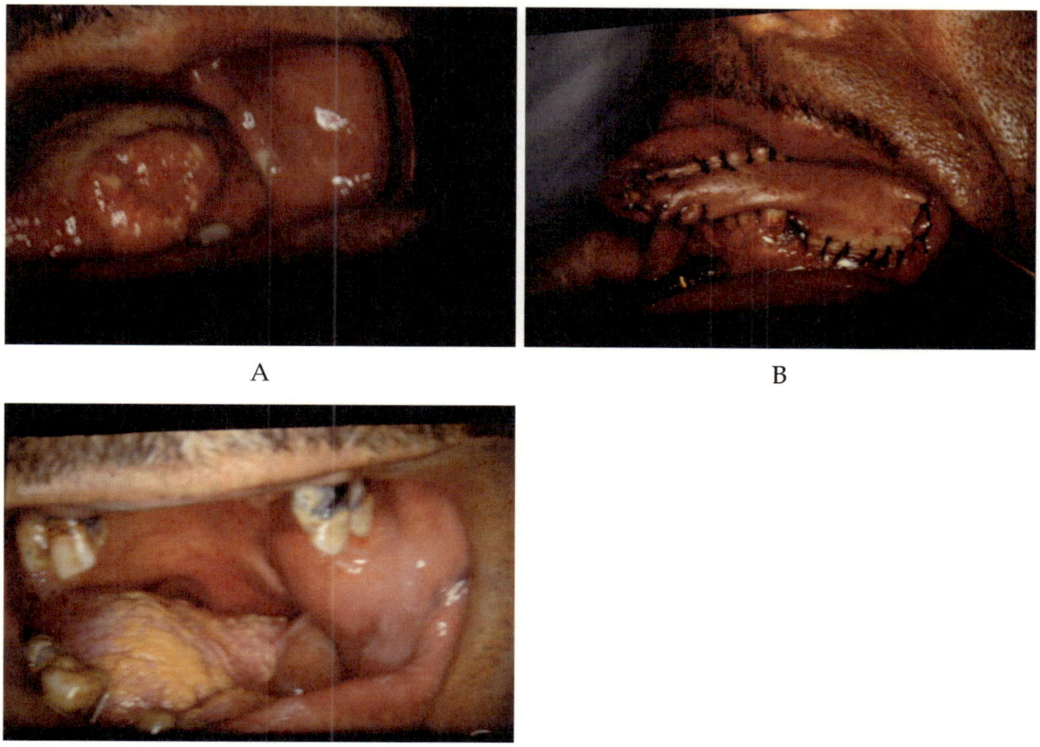

A B

C

Fig. 5. Reconstruction of the tongue by LCF. A-Squamous cell carcinoma of the lateral side of the tongue, B-Immediate reconstruction of the tongue by LCF after hemiglosactomy, C- Three years post operative photograph showing excellent reconstruction of the tongue after hemi glosactomy

3. Reconstruction by LCF of peri oral tissue in cases with post traumatic missile injuries

In 10 cases LCF was used for reconstruction of the lip and sub-mental area after excision of scars in the region to advance the chin and sub mental area upward and to make a room for reconstruction of the lost part of the mandible by bone graft from the iliac crest as a good donor area for bone grafting to get good bulk, rigidity, shape and good amount of cancellous bone. Reconstruction of the lip by fan rotation flap also the flap been used for reconstruction of large missing part of the lip. The results of these cases were quiet good. 1,3,4

4. The use of platysma muscle flap for reconstruction of atrophied masseter muscle

In this technique platysma muscle was used by the author for reconstruction of the atrophied masseter muscle in cases with mild hemi facial micro somia or first arch dysplasia syndrome,4 cases were treated by this technique and the result quiet good.

Complications of LCV:

1. Oro cutanous fistula:

The complication of LCF in reconstruction of intra oral defect is the oro cutanous fistula, which represent a tunnel for introducing the flap proper of LCV to the oral cavity for reconstruction of the cheek, floor of the mouth, tongue or alveolus, this fistula usually closed within 6 weeks and the orifice of the tunnel usually closed by iodoform pak to prevent saliva and fluid leakage. This situation is very un pleasant to the patient but we have to assure the patient about this matter and only a temporary situation. To enhance healing and closure of the fistula we usually de squamate the skin of the fistula. These fistula occurred in all cases with intra oral defect and required reconstruction by LCF and been used in 23 cases.

2. Flap necrosis:

Necrosis was reported by the author in the terminal part of the LCV specially in the floor of the mouth and the tongue due to accumulation of food and fluid, these cases was controlled by Lavage with improvement of oral hygien.this condition was reported in 4 cases and healed very quickly after 2 weeks.

3. Infection:

Infection reported in 3 cases due to food debries.These condition was treated by Lavage and proper dis infecting mouth wash and proper anti biotic.

Evolution of Lateral Cervical Flap (LCF):

It is thought that LCV an excellent flap introduced by the author and advocated before 2 decades for reconstruction of the floor of the oral cavity, the tongue, alveoulus of the lower jaw and the cheek. , 1These sites the most common for involvement by oral cancer. The work published in 1994 as a preliminary report, 2. Reconstruction of these anatomical sites was a problem for many surgeons and for many years during the last 4 decades in the last century. Tube pedicle flap was the most popular and probably the only flap used for reconstruction ,the objection about tube pedicle is a long surgical procedure required many steps during transfer as secondary stage from the abdomen before been used for orofacial region reconstruction, the procedure takes many months till reconstruction, the color of skin of the abdomen does not match the color of skin of orofacial and the whole procedure with<delay technique> no more accepted for reconstruction of the face. Introduction of temporal flap by McGregor in the early 1960s did a great contribution to science and a great advance to cancer surgery of the head and neck.Disadvanttage of this technique is a 2 stage operation and flap transfer and successful reconstruction of the oral cavity were annoying to the patients because of growing hair in the mouth. The author did shaving the hair to please his patients and the area look rather bulky with deformity of the forhead.Many other good flaps advocated before and during that time such as deltoid pectoral flap of Bakamijian and Ariyan with his pectorals major myocutanous flap. All these flaps showed good result in reconstruction of the oral cavity, but the dis advantages about deltoid pectoral flap, being a random flap and not recommended for older people because of atherosclerosis of the blood vessels and a 2 stage operation, a pectorals major flap required a long distance transfer and the size of the tissue is limited and not suitable for large defect reconstruction in the oral cavity and recommended for intra oral or extra oral small defect, also the color of the chest does not match the color of the face

Free flap surgery is an excellent flap like forearm flap advocated by the Chinese surgeons in the early seventies of the last century for reconstruction of the orofacial regions, but this procedure required skill and highly trained in micro vascular anastomosis and it is a time consuming procedure and the skin transferred does not match the skin of orofacial region in addition the possibilities of failure due to thrombosis of the vessels.1,2,3,4

The superiority of LCF proved to be an excellent axial flap and an excellent technique for reconstruction of perioral and oral cavity both in radical cancer surgery of the mouth and for reconstruction of sub mental area in post traumatic missile injuries of the face as a one stage operation,3 and further to that the skin of the side of the neck match the texture and color of the face with quick healing due to high vascularity of the flap. The thickness of the flap is well tolerated by the oral cavity and no hair growing from the flap.

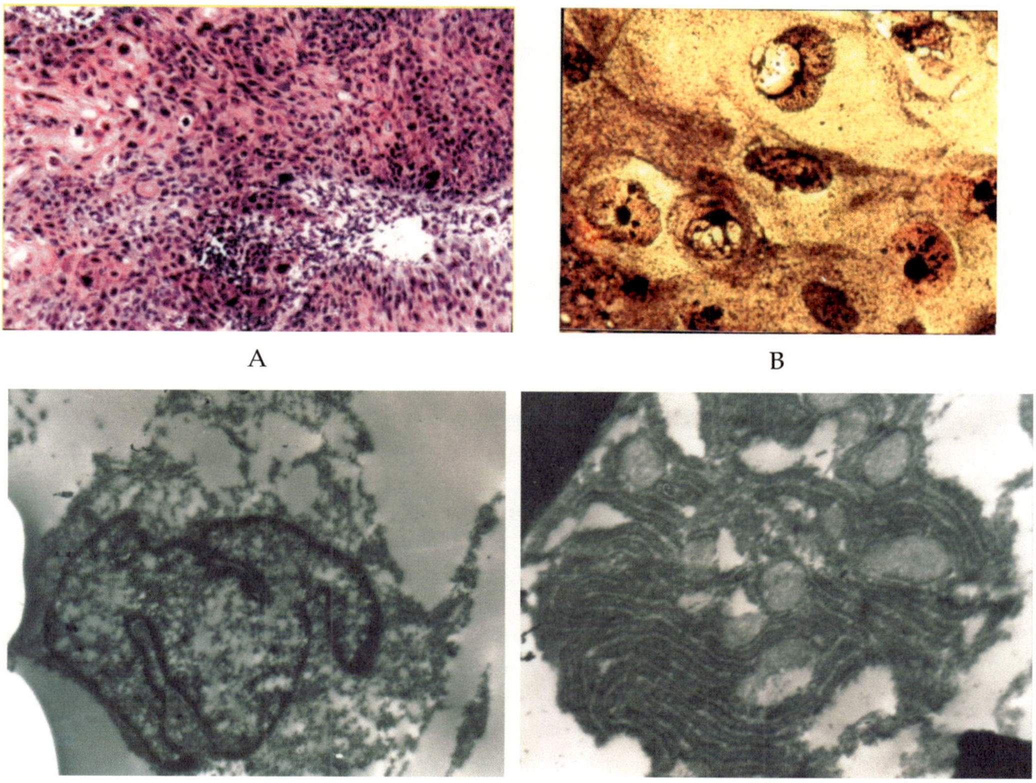

Fig. 6. Study of proliferative activity of squamous cell carcinoma. A-Poorly differentiated squamous cell carcinoma of the oral cavity (H&E X40), B-AgNOR staining of poorly differentiated squamous cell carcinoma showing the number of dot of NOR increased in the cell due to high proliferative activity of the cells, high magnification, C- High magnification of single cell of poorly differentiated squamous cell carcinoma showing nucleus of the cell divided into many nucleuses (EM X 36000), D-High magnification by electron microscopy of poorly differentiated squamous cell carcinoma showing high proliferative activity of endoplasmic reticulum with many mitochondria in between (EM X36000)

The flap design and its elevation make a good access for radical resection of the mandible with supra hyoid neck dissection and without using the flap for reconstruction, and the type of incisions used and after reconstruction does not leave a long vertical band of scar tissue extend from upper neck down to the clavicle region has been observed by the author with other techniques.

5. Acknowledgments

I would like to thank Professor Mutaz Habal editor J Craniofacial Surgery for his kind permission to use illustrations and figures from my paper entitled (Reconstruction by lateral cervical flap of peri oral and oral cavity….) 2010, Vol 21; 3 and to Jahn Nesland ,editor of J Ultra structural Pathology and Informa Health care for permission to use Fig.6 from my paper entitled (Proliferative activity in oral carcinoma ….) 2008, Vol 32;137-144 and special appreciation to Ms Alenka Urbancic,editor production of Neck Dissection book and In Tech-Open Access publisher for their kind assistant and help.

6. References

[1] Kummoona R: Reconstruction by lateral cervical flap of perioral and oral cavity: clinical and experimental studies' Craniofacial Surg., 2010, 21, number 3

[2] Kummoona R: Use of lateral cervical flap in the reconstructive surgery of the orofacial region.Int.J.Oral Maxillofacial.Surg.1994, 23; 85-89

[3] Kummoona R: Posttrumatic missile injuries of the orofacial region Craniofacial Surg.2008,19;300-305

[4] Kummoona R:Reconstruction of the mandible and oral cavity after tumor surgery.In:Karcher H,Zwitting P,eds.Functional Surgery of the Head &Neck; Proceeding of the First International Meeting of the Head&Neck.Graz Druck and Verlagsanastalt,1989;197-199

[5] Kummoona R,Jabbar A,AL-Rahal D K:Proliferative activity in oral carcinoma; studied with Ag-NOR and electron microscopy.Ultrastructural Pathol 2008;32:137-144

[6] Kummoona R: The managements of orofacial tumors of children in Iraq Craniofacial Surgery.2009,20;143-50

[7] Kummoona R: The use of EM for studding Apoptotic changes and Proliferative Activity of Oral Carcinoma and Jaw Lymphoma. In A Mendez-Vilas& J Diaz,eds. Microscopy Science, Technology, Application and Education, CFORMATEX, 2010;52-65

[8] Kummoona R: Periorbital and orbital malignancies: Methods of managements and reconstruction inIraq.Craniofacial Surgery.2007,18;1370-75

[9] Kummoona R: Reconstruction of the mandible by bone graft and metal prosthesis.2009, 20; 1100-1107

[10] Kummoona R,Sami S M,Al Kapptan I,Al Muala H.Study of anti apoptotic gene of oral carcinoma by using Bcl2 oncogene.J Oral Pathol Med.2007,37;345-51

6

Advanced Developments in Neck Dissection Technique: Perspectives in Minimally Invasive Surgery

Jandee Lee and Woong Youn Chung
Department of Surgery, Yonsei Univeristy College of Medicine
South Korea

1. Introduction

Over the last decade, surgeons have experienced dramatic changes in operative procedures as a result of the development of remarkable new technological tools that have enabled significant advances in minimally invasive surgical techniques and instruments. These advances have led to the increased application of minimally invasive techniques for "non-conventional" procedures. The potential benefits of minimally invasive surgery have included reduced levels of trauma to the tissues, decreased postoperative pain, reduced length of hospital stay, and better cosmetic outcomes. Various types of minimally invasive operative techniques have been introduced, including mini-incision, video-assisted, endoscopic, robotic, laparoendoscopic single-site surgery (LESS), and natural orifice trans-luminal endoscopic surgery (NOTES™). In head and neck surgery, where vital structures are in close proximity to each other, and the operative field is a deep and narrow space, these minimally invasive approaches can be especially challenging. Minimally invasive surgery is not minimum surgery, and the principle of complete tumor resection must still be followed. Therefore, head and neck surgeons have often avoided minimally invasive techniques due to concerns about visualization, damage to vital structures, and limited availability of instruments specific to the delicate tasks required of the head and neck surgeon.

Minimally invasive neck surgery through totally endoscopic or video-assisted techniques, which are currently being used around the globe for thyroid and parathyroid surgeries, enables a smaller wound size or allows for the positioning of the wound in areas of cosmetic benefit. Since Michel Gagner first described endoscopic neck surgery in 1996, endoscopic procedures based on various approaches have been widely applied. In addition to minimized scarring and improved cosmetic results, the adoption of endoscopic procedures has offered several extra advantages, such as diminished postoperative hyperesthesia or paresthesia of the anterior neck and less patient discomfort during swallowing, which may sometimes result from the conventional transverse cervical incision. However even with these potential advantages, the technical limitations of endoscopic neck surgery, which are shared by many other types of minimally invasive surgery, have remained a significant consideration. The skills required in using straight, rigid endoscopic instruments without articulations and a two-dimensional (2D) view are radically different from those applied in the 3D milieu of conventional surgery performed directly by the surgeon's expert hands. Furthermore, particularly in the head and neck area, the workspace during endoscopic surgery is narrow and restrictive. Although several minimally invasive techniques have been adopted in the attempt to avoid long cervical scars, purely endoscopic methods have been technically limited when procedures are complex.

In many fields, surgeons have introduced robotic techniques to minimally invasive procedures and have gradually overcome such limitations. The new da Vinci S surgical robot system (Intuitive, Inc., Sunnyvale, CA) is increasingly available, and because of the complexities of certain laparoscopic procedures, the extended capabilities offered by this robotic technology are gaining wide acceptance. The da Vinci S system allows operations to be performed more safely and meticulously than conventional endoscopic procedures by providing a 3D, magnified, and stable operative view. Head and neck surgeons have begun to incorporate surgical robotics in minimally invasive neck surgery to overcome the constraints observed during endoscopic surgery. In head and neck surgery, robotic techniques permit better visualization and a wider range of manipulations that can fit in a deep and narrow space. The authors have recently reported our initial experience with 33 patients who underwent modified radical neck dissection using robotic techniques. The results seem promising, with greater surgical scope and no serious complications.

In this chapter, we introduce the newly developed technologies in neck surgery and evaluate how some of these developments might improve surgical outcomes. These advanced technologies include the development of various endoscopic techniques, and the da Vinci robot surgical system.

2. Minimally invasive neck dissection

2.1 History of neck dissection

The first documented neck dissection was performed in 1888 by Franciszek Jawdynski, but the first description of neck dissection technique was presented by George Crile in 1906. Since then, neck dissection has evolved into a more refined set of procedures that allow for a greater degree of conservation and reduced morbidity. This modern technique, radical block dissection of all the deep lymphatic structures in the neck, has been described in detail (Rinaldo et al, 2008). Radical neck dissection in a series of 132 patients was found to have a mortality rate of 8% and a 3-year survival rate of 38% (Kazi, 2003); however 86 of these 132 patients underwent types of dissection that likely corresponded to modern selective neck dissections rather than en bloc radical neck dissection. Following a report showing the results of 665 operations in 599 patients by Martin et al. (1951), the technique of Martin, similar in most respects to that of Crile, became the standard "radical neck dissection", and for many years was considered the only truly curative procedure for regional lymph node disease in patients with head and neck cancer. This operation involved the removal of all lymphatic and non-lymphatic structures from the mandible to the clavicle and between the platysma and the prevertebral fascia, except for the carotid arteries; hypoglossal, lingual, vagus and phrenic nerves; and brachial plexus. The lateral boundary of the dissection was the anterior border of the trapezius muscle, and the medial border was the midline of the neck, superficial to the infrahyoid muscles, and the opposite digastric muscle superficial to the suprahyoid (mylohyoid) muscle (Ferlito et al, 2009). A standard selective neck dissection that spares the spinal accessory nerve was also described (Ward & Robben, 1951). At that time, the technique of neck dissection included the en-bloc resection of the spinal accessory nerve, the jugular vein and the sternocleidomastoid muscle, and in some cases, the resection of the vagus nerve. This method, however, was not widely accepted until the 1980s, when studies comparing radical and modified radical neck dissections revealed similar oncologic results but more compromised function and greater shoulder pain for patients who underwent radical neck procedures. This change in extent of surgery had an important impact on elective neck dissection, maximizing the use of a preventive treatment that is less invasive but that does not diminish oncologic results (Kowalski & Sanabria, 2007).

2.2 Classification of neck dissection

2.2.1 Neck node nomenclature and classification

Over the past decade, the nomenclature and classification of neck dissection have not changed; if anything, they have become more simplified and standardized. According to the revised neck dissection classification proposed by the American Head and Neck Society and the American Academy of Otolaryngology–Head and Neck Surgery (AAO-HNS), the lymph nodes of the neck are divided into six levels (I–VI) (Robbins et al, 2001) (Table 1) (Figure 1).
In 2008, the Committee for Neck Dissection Classification of the AHNS prepared a contemporary revision, to keep classifications consistent with current practice (Robbins et al, 2008). Now that imaging modalities are used in staging the neck, radiologic landmarks are needed to define the boundaries between lymph node levels. This classification system, however, has given rise to several concerns (Ferlito et al, 2008). First, the boundary that separates sublevels IB and IIA is currently defined as the border of the stylohyoid muscle.

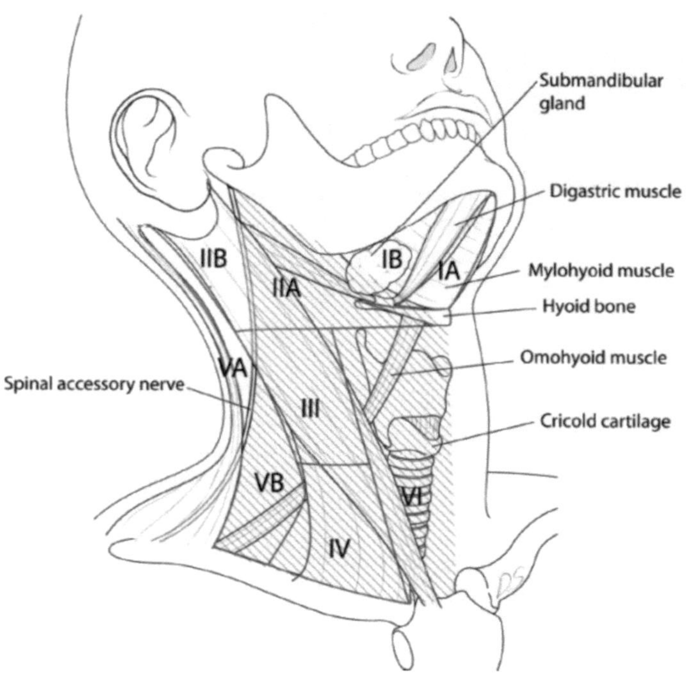

Fig. 1. Anatomic landmarks used to divide the lateral and central lymph node compartments into levels I-VI; the area with a peculiar fold line is where lymph node dissection is made during radical neck dissection (Kang et al, 2011).

Neck node level	Superior boundary	Inferior boundary	Anteromedial boundary	Posterolateral boundary
IA (submental)	Symphysis of mandible	Body of hyoid	Anterior belly of contralateral digastric muscle	Anterior belly of ipsilateral digastric muscle
IB (submandibular)	Body of mandible	Posterior belly of digastric muscle	Anterior belly of digastric muscle	Stylohyoid muscle
IIA (upper jugular)	Skull base	Horizontal plane defined by the inferior body of the hyoid bone	Stylohyoid muscle	Vertical plane defined by the spinal accessory nerve
IIB (upper jugular)	Skull base	Horizontal plane defined by the inferior body of the hyoid bone	Vertical plane defined by the spinal accessory nerve	Lateral border of the sternocleidomastoid muscle
III (middle jugular)	Horizontal plane defined by the inferior body of the hyoid bone	Horizontal plane defined by the inferior border of the cricoid cartilage	Lateral border of the sternohyoid muscle	Lateral border of the sternocleidomastoid muscle
IV (lower jugular)	Horizontal plane defined by the inferior border of the cricoid cartilage	Clavicle	Lateral border of the sternohyoid muscle	Lateral border of the sternocleidomastoid muscle
VA (posterior triangle)	Apex of convergence of the sternocleidomastoid and trapezius muscle	Horizontal plane defined by the inferior border of the cricoid cartilage	Posterior border of the sternocleidomastoid muscle	Anterior border of the trapezius muscle
VB (posterior triangle)	Horizontal plane defined by the inferior border of the cricoid cartilage	Clavicle	Posterior border of the sternocleidomastoid muscle	Anterior border of the trapezius muscle
VI (anterior compartment)	Hyoid bone	Suprasternal	Common carotid artery	Common carotid artery

Table 1. Lymph node nomenclature and classification in neck dissection (Robbins et al, 2002)

While this anatomical landmark can be recognized during neck dissection, it is difficult to determine during physical examination or on imaging modalities. Therefore, the Committee proposed that the border between levels I and II be the vertical plane defined by the posterior edge of the submandibular gland, that the boundary between levels II and III be the hyoid bone, and the boundary between levels III and IV be the cricoid cartilage. Level VI is currently defined as lying below the body of the hyoid bone, above the top of the manubrium, and between the lateral borders of the sternohyoid muscles, which separate level VI from levels II and III. However, the sternohyoid muscles are not easy to define radiologically. Thus, the Committee proposed that the lateral borders of level VI be defined as the inner margins of the carotid arteries, which in most patients can be easily palpated as well as viewed radiologically (Ferlito et al, 2008).

According to the neck node classification of the AHNS, both lymph nodes of the superior mediastinum (often referred to as level VII) and lymph nodes outside the neck groupings (i.e. the retropharyngeal, periparotid, and buccinator nodes) are not included in this classification, but are designated by their specific group. Although the superior mediastinal lymph nodes have been referred to as "level VII," the Neck Dissection Classification Committee of the AHNS does not recommend use of this term, as it defines a region outside the typical boundaries of the neck. The Committee has sought to prevent the establishment of new levels defining other lymph node groups, thus avoiding a more complex numbering system (Ferlito et al, 2008). However, the term level VII continues to be employed in many publications to represent the lymph nodes in the superior mediastinal group. Thus, the new Committee recommends that level VII refer to the extension of the chain of paratracheal nodes below the suprasternal notch (the dividing line between levels VI and VII) to the level of the innominate artery only. As an alternative to naming this group level VII, these nodes may be designated as "the superior mediastinal lymph nodes, above the level of the innominate artery." This level is defined by the sternal notch superiorly and the innominate artery inferiorly, landmarks that are readily identifiable on imaging modalities. The Committee noted that nodes in level VII are usually accessible through the cervical incision. Mediastinal lymph nodes inferior to the innominate artery require sternotomy for access, and are not included in level VII (Robbins et al, 2008).

2.2.2 Neck dissection classification

The updated American Joint Committee on Cancer (AJCC) staging system has highlighted the significance of the biology of lymph node metastases and has refined selective neck dissection procedures by correlating surgical with radiologic landmarks, thus facilitating multidisciplinary cooperation among surgeons, radiologists and oncologists. The currently employed definitions of neck dissection terminology and definitions and indications for types of selective node dissection are shown in Table 2 (Ferlito et al, 2009).

Several types of neck dissection have been described. Radical neck dissection consists of levels I–V with the associated sternocleidomastoid muscle, jugular vein and spinal accessory nerve. Modified radical neck dissection consists of levels I–V without any of the aforementioned non-lymphatic structures. Selective neck dissection consists of any dissection that excludes one or more lymph node levels included in a radical neck dissection (i.e. levels II–IV). Extended neck dissection includes one or more additional lymph node groups or nonlymphatic structures in addition to those of a radical neck dissection, including periparotid lymph nodes and parotidectomy or superior mediastinal nodes and level VI.

The purpose of neck dissection may be therapeutic, to treat lymph node metastases found during a physical or imaging examination; opportune, when the approach for exposure and

Terminology	Extent of neck dissection
Radical neck dissection	Removal of lymph nodes levels I-V sternocleidomastoid muscle, spinal accessory nerve, and internal jugular vein.
Modified neck dissection	Removal of lymph nodes levels I-M (as in radical neck dissection), but preservation of at least one of the non-lymphatic structures (sternocleidomastoid muscle, spinal accessory nerve, and internal jugular vein). Each non-lymphatic structure that is removed should be named.
Selective neck dissection	Preservation of one or more lymph node levels relative to a radical neck dissection.
Extended neck dissection	Removal of an additional lymph node level or group or a non-lymphatic structure relative to a radical neck dissection (muscle, blood vessel, nerve). An example of other lymph node groups can be – superior mediastinal, parapharyngeal, retropharyngeal, peri-parotid, postauricular, suboccipital, or buccinators. An example of other non-lymphatic structure can be external carotid artery, hypoglossal or vagus nerves.

Table 2. Definitions of neck dissection (Ferlito et al, 2009)

resection of a malignant primary tumor is through the neck; or elective, when lymph node compromise is not found clinically or by imaging, but the risk of microscopic metastases is higher than the risk associated with an additional surgical procedure and its attendant morbidity. In principle, indications for neck dissection in oral cancer patients must include a risk-benefit analysis, balancing the probabilities of neck metastases, complications associated with neck dissection and the possible prognostic influence of late diagnosis of metastasis during follow-up. If the probability of neck metastases is high, neck dissection with its intrinsic morbidity has the same effect as therapeutic dissection, decreasing the risk of regional recurrence. However, if the probability of neck metastases is low or nil, neck dissection is an overtreatment, with morbidities arising from the neck procedure possibly resulting in a reduced quality of life and increased functional deficits. Although this risk-benefit analysis would yield better results if it were possible to predict the risk of neck metastases, this type of prediction is difficult to introduce and apply in clinical practice (Kowalski & Sanabria, 2007).

Due to the development of a variety of surgical procedures for managing regional disease in head and neck cancer, a system of classification has evolved. Once it was demonstrated that standard radical neck dissection was not necessary for effective management of cervical metastatic disease in all patients, the procedures were modified and the extent and location of dissection altered to conform to the proven or surmised lymph node levels at risk. This has resulted in a plethora of procedures that have become increasingly difficult to name and classify. The currently employed classification system has built on previous definitions of node levels and types of neck dissection. Nevertheless, the many permutations of possible levels and structures removed have made it difficult to describe the type of resection in each patient. This system, however, has the advantages of familiar terminology and definitions, thus facilitating its employment (Ferlito et al, 2009).

2.3 Distribution of neck metastasis from various primary sites and extent of neck dissection

Neck node metastasis is the most important prognostic factor in patients with several types of head and neck carcinoma, making the management of neck metastases in head and neck cancer one of the most important aspects of treatment. Although therapeutic neck dissection has been found to affect the prognosis of head and neck cancer patients, the role of elective neck dissection remains unclear. Of head and neck malignancies, oral cancer has been the most widely assessed using elective neck dissection. However, the amount and quality of information currently available cannot definitively determine the prognostic effects of elective neck dissection. Furthermore, the recent introduction of sentinel lymph node biopsy in the diagnosis and treatment of head and neck cancer has suggested that elective neck dissection may not be clinically useful (Kowalski & Sanabria, 2007).

The idea of removing individual node levels immediately draining the primary cancer site originated during the 19th century. Supraomohyoid neck dissection (node levels I–III) for oral and oropharyngeal cancer, jugular chain neck dissection (levels II–IV) for laryngeal cancer, and central compartment node dissection (level VI) for thyroid cancer were performed later, mostly in patients with clinically negative necks, but these procedures were considered to be of benefit mainly for staging purposes (Ferlito et al, 2009). The major therapeutic advance in the past two decades has been the refinement of the various selective neck dissections to achieve oncologic control and minimize morbidity. These selective dissections can be tailored to individual patients to some extent since there is now an awareness of the pattern of spread for each head and neck site. Table 3 summarizes the lymph node levels likely to be involved (and thus included in a selective dissection) based on site (Seethala et al, 2009).

Primary tumor site	Lymphatic drainage pattern
Oral cavity	Level I – III (sometimes IV)
Oropharynx, hypopharynx, larynx	Levels II-IV (IIA only for some Squamous cell carcinoma of larynx and hypopharynx)
Larynx with subglottic involvement	Levels IV-VI
Thyroid	Level VI (level II-V if level V is clinically +)

Table 3. Common drainage patterns for tumors of various head and neck sites (Robbins et al, 2002)

2.4 Minimally invasive neck dissection

2.4.1 Minimally invasive video-assisted neck dissection

There have been only a few reports on a minimally invasive approach for neck dissection. During thyroid surgery, modified radical neck dissection is usually performed through a large transverse incision (extended collar incision). In some patients, an additional McFee incision may be necessary to clear neck level II. Video assisted thyroidectomy therefore became a valid option for patients with thyroid nodules and low risk papillary thyroid carcinomas. In addition, video assisted central neck lymph node dissection was shown to be feasible in patients with papillary thyroid carcinoma (Bellantone et al, 2002), resulting in the development of a minimally invasive video-assisted lateral neck dissection approach

(VALNED) (Lombardi et al, 2007). This type of surgery begins by making a 4 cm cervical incision between the cricoid cartilage and sternal notch. A 30° endoscope (5 mm) is used for better vision and the operating field is exposed by retractors. Under visual control the neck dissection is performed with conventional instruments, although use of a harmonic scalpel is preferred. The mean number of nodes removed per side was 25. The cosmetic results of the 4 cm horizontal incision were superior to those of conventional approaches. Although VALNED is a safe and feasible technique, additional studies are needed to show that the completeness of resection is similar to that of conventional open approaches.

2.4.2 Endoscopic neck dissection

The outcomes of minimally invasive video assisted thyroidectomies have suggested that endoscopic techniques have advantages for other types of head and neck surgery. The relatively longer operation time using this approach is likely due to the narrower operative field and the presence of many vital structures in the neck. Although endoscopic operations were initially limited to regions with natural cavities such as the peritoneum and pleura, the use of endoscopic approaches for head and neck surgery has extended their indications to regions without a natural cavity. All validated methods try to reduce the extent of surgical trauma and its associated morbidity (Muenscher et al, 2011). The main reasons for the development of endoscopic neck surgery are the unpredictable risks of unsatisfactory cosmetic results. For patients with benign neck lesions, this would mean replacing one deformity with another. Further, use of endoscopic methods results in faster wound healing and reduced morbidity due to complications.

Ten endoscopic neck dissections on five human cadavers showed that the majority of neck lymph nodes could be removed by this approach (Dulguerov et al, 2001). Endoscopic selective neck dissection has been utilized in a porcine model (Terris et al, 2003), and endoscopic neck surgery with lymph node dissection has been performed on patients with thyroid neoplasms (Kitagawa et al, 2003; Miccoli & Materazzi, 2004). Gasless skin lifting techniques, approaching lateral neck levels during thyroidectomy, have also been performed (Kitagawa et al, 2003). The results of endoscopic lymph node excisions in patients with squamous cell carcinomas of the upper aerodigestive tract located at different sites (uvula, epiglottis and glottis), as well as those of endoscopic sentinel lymphadenectomy for diagnosis of the N0 neck, were presented in 2004 (Werner et al, 2004). It is unclear whether the N0 neck in surgically treated head and neck carcinomas should be accessed by neck dissection or regular clinical follow up, although an endoscopic approach may be an alternative to tracer uptake by sentinel lymph nodes. A small skin incision chosen for endoscopy may be extended for standard neck dissection. In this method, a rigid endoscope is introduced through a specially designed tube, allowing the labeled lymph node to be dissected after removing subcutaneous adipose tissue. The sentinel node concept combines endoscopic lymph node dissection with frozen section analysis to explore the N0 neck. Alternatively, an approach called stealth surgery can be used for transaxillary subcutaneous endoscopic excision of benign neck lesions (Dutta et al, 2008). This endoscopic method may reduce the degree of invasiveness frequently associated with sentinel lymphadenectomy. A recent editorial concluded that "It will take a lot of work before we know if endoscopic neck dissection is a good, oncologic operation, but the trip to learn such a truth should be interesting" (Richtsmeier, 2003). At present, however, this procedure has not achieved widespread acceptance in clinical practice (Ferlito et al, 2006).

2.4.3 Characteristics of endoscopic approaches for neck surgery

In general, it is important to distinguish between two approaches for neck dissection. In one, a pure endoscopic approach is use to insert ports and to achieve a working space correlating with visceral or non-visceral organs by insufflating gas/air. The instruments are inserted through special trocars. In the second, minimally invasive approach, such as video-assisted approaches, skin incisions are larger, and the working space is maintained by external retraction of the skin. In these approaches, the endoscope is a means to improve the view through a small opening. In both approaches, dissection is usually performed "conventionally", often by using a harmonic scalpel. All of these procedures are designed to reduce the extent of surgical trauma and morbidity and were established during surgery for complete removal of involved organs. However, there have been few descriptions of neck dissections and standard procedures have not yet been established.

Typically, neck lesions are removed through skin incisions. Some horizontal incisions may be made to blend with skin creases. However, other surgical scars on the face and neck may become hypertrophic or keloid scars, having a lifelong impact on patients. Endoscopic approaches may produce smaller scars, by making small incisions in areas easy to hide (e.g. the axilla). Video assisted or gasless axillary procedures still require larger skin incisions, but the retraction and improved overview provided by the endoscope can significantly reduce incision size, while allowing easy extension of these incisions in patients switched to open procedures. The major disadvantage of these techniques is prolonged operation time, which, however, can be shortened as surgeons become more experienced. Table 4 describes the advantages and disadvantages of endoscopic and video-assisted approaches with or without gas.

Gas insufflation technique	
Advantages	Smallest incisions (Ports) Best cosmetic results Shorter time in hospital
Disadvantages	Arterial injury Venous injury Embolism Pneumothroax Pneumomediastinum Subcutaneous emphysema Special training Special equipment Prolonged operation time
Gasless technique (flap retraction technique)	
Advantages	Single incisions Magnified operating field Good cosmetic results Short time in hospital Easy to convert approach Possibility use of microscope
Disadvantages	Limited tumor size Retraction affects wounds Prolonged operation time

Table 4. Advantages and disadvantages of various endoscopic techniques. (Muenscher et al, 2011)

Furthermore, endoscopic and minimally invasive/video assisted dissections require special instruments and are more costly and time consuming. Although complication rates are low after endoscopic neck surgery, several morbidities, such as injuries to arteries and veins, embolism, subcutaneous emphysema, pneumothorax and pneumomediastinum, were described in early reports on the use of these methods in thyroid surgery. Many of these complications, however, may have been due to gas insufflation to enhance working space. Moreover, as in any other type of endoscopic surgery, common surgical complications, such as nerve injury and wound infection, can occur. These complications depend on patient selection, especially since indications for minimally invasive approaches have not been determined. Conversion to open procedures is common in oncologic settings such as proven N+ status in patients with head and neck carcinomas. To date, there have been no prospective randomized clinical trials comparing open with endoscopic or video assisted surgery, especially regarding the extent of resection. Minimally invasive approaches are advantageous for patients with benign neck lesions, thyroid disease, and selective/sentinel lymph node dissections, due to better cosmetic results and shorter wound healing times. Surgeons tend to favor video assisted minimally invasive techniques or endoscopic surgery using a gasless transaxillary approach, creating the working space by retraction, because the gas filling procedures, especially at level IV, bear some risks (Muenscher et al, 2011).

2.5 Robot technique for head and neck cancer

The endoscopic technique represents a considerable technologic advance and has recently been applied to head and neck surgery. Several trials of endoscopic neck surgery plus radical node dissection in patients with head and neck as well as thyroid cancer have shown that the endoscopic approach to neck dissection eliminates the long cervical scar. Furthermore, to overcome displeasing cosmetic outcomes, several endoscopic approaches to neck dissection have been conducted using remote skin incision. However, endoscopic surgery is more demanding and requires more time than open surgery, primarily because of instrumental and anatomical limitations. The instruments used to perform these minimally invasive endoscopic surgeries have definite limitations such as a 2-dimensional flat monitor, rigid and straight endoscopic instruments, and no tactile sense. Endoscopic surgery is particularly problematic for complex and difficult procedures such as radical neck dissection for head and neck cancer, in keeping with the principles of oncologic safety. The da Vinci surgical robot system (Intuitive Surgical, Sunnyvale, CA, USA) was developed to overcome these limitations (Chung et al, 2011). This surgical robot system promises more precise, improved endoscopic techniques and enables compartment-oriented anatomical neck dissection. Moreover, the robotic technique for minimally invasive surgery has other advantages, including the increased dexterity of the instrumentation used. Use of the robot system in head and neck surgery eliminates some of the technical pitfalls and limitations of endoscopic surgery. Furthermore, advances in robotic techniques, such as a steady camera platform, a 3-dimensional magnified operative view, 7 degrees of freedom, scaled and tremor-filtered movements, and a multi-articulated endo-wrist, allow precise and complex endoscopic procedures to be performed. Accordingly, the meticulous and precise motions of modern robotic instruments have introduced new levels of technical safety and feasibility to robotic thyroidectomy.

We recently described 33 patients who underwent robotic modified radical neck dissection using a gasless transaxillary approach, and provided details of operative techniques and short-term operative outcomes (Kang et al, 2011). To our knowledge, this was the first report of robotic radical neck dissection technique in head and neck surgery. We found that the short-term operative outcomes were satisfactory, with no serious postoperative complications. This technique allowed precise manipulation of robotic instruments and complete compartment-oriented dissection without injuring major vessels or nerves or compromising surgical oncologic principles. Moreover, esthetic outcomes were maximized by using a remote axillary incision site, allowing the incision scar in the axilla to be completely concealed when the arm is down in its natural position, with the small anterior chest wall incision scar becoming almost inconspicuous over time (see Figure 2 & 3).

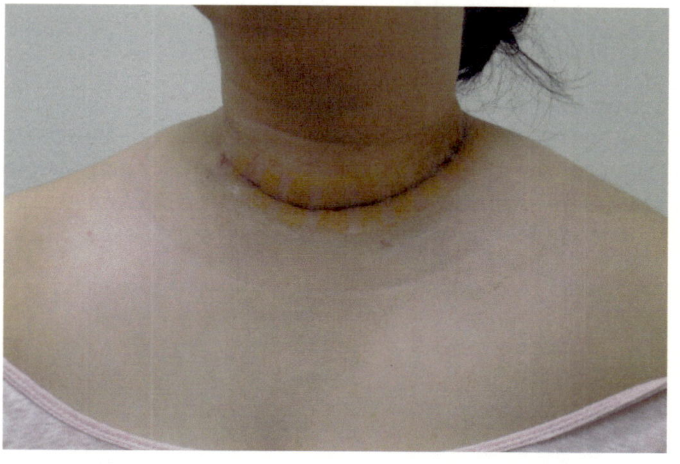

Fig. 2. Photograph of a postoperative scar with an extended long collar incision after conventional open modified radical neck dissection.

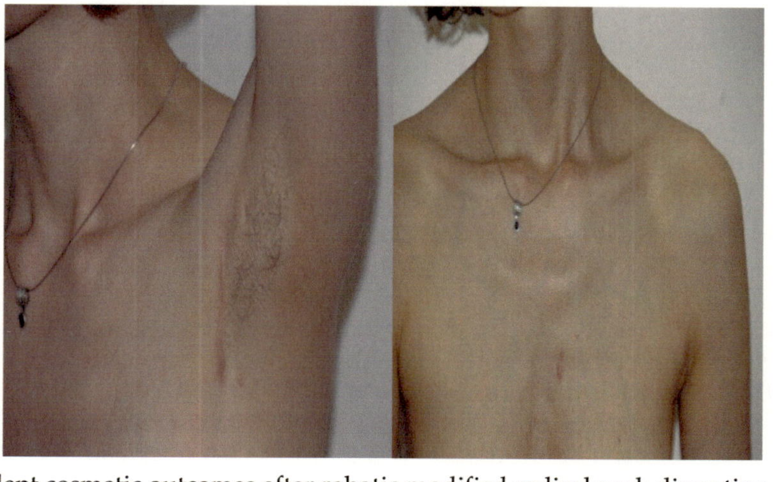

Fig. 3. Excellent cosmetic outcomes after robotic modified radical neck dissection. The long axillary scar is concealed when the patient's arm is by her side in the normal position, and most of the small anterior chest wall scar eventually becomes inconspicuous several months after the operation.

However, robotic neck dissection for patients with head-and-neck cancer remains at an early stage, and many unanswered questions remain; the benefits afforded by the technique require further evaluation.

2.6 Robotic neck dissection technique

In robotic modified radical neck dissection technique, the complete anatomical neck lymph node dissection, matching that of the open method, was found to be possible using excellent robotic instruments, such as magnified and 3-dimensional operative field, a stable camera platform, multi-articulated and tremor filtering system, and three accessible robotic arms. We briefly introduced our robotic modified radical neck dissection technique (Kang et al, 2011).

2.6.1 Operative set-up and creation of working space

With the patient in the supine positions and under general anesthesia, the neck is is extended slightly by inserting a soft pillow under the shoulder and the face is turned away from the lesion. The lesion side arm is abducted to expose axilla and lateral neck, and the head is tilted and rotated to face the non-lesion side (Fig. 4).

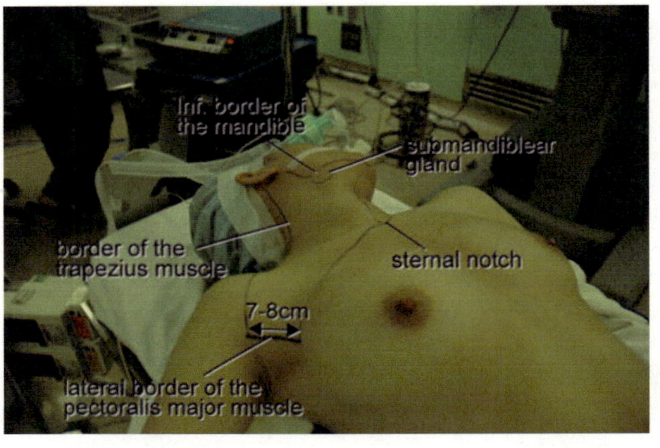

Fig. 4. Patient position for robotic modified radical neck dissection using a gasless transaxillary approach (Chung et al, 2011).

The landmarks for flap dissection are bounded by the sternal notch and the midline of the anterior neck medially, the anterior border of the trapezius muscle laterally, and the submandibular gland superiorly.

A 7-8cm vertical skin incision is placed in the axilla along the anterior axillary fold and the lateral border of the pectoralis major muscle. The subcutaneous flap from the axilla to the midline of the anterior neck is dissected over the anterior surface of the pectoralis major muscle and clavicle by electrical cautery under direct vision. After exposing the clavicle, subplatysmal flap dissection proceeds to the midline of the anterior neck medially, to the upper point where the external jugular vein and greater auricular nerve cross the lateral border of the sternocleidomastoid (SCM) muscle superiorly. The external jugular vein is ligated at the crossing point of the SCM muscle. Laterally the trapezius muscle is identified and dissected upwards along its anterior border. During the flap dissection in the posterior neck area, the spinal accessory nerve is identified and exposed along its course. After subplatysmal flap dissection, the clavicular head of the SCM is divided at the level of its attachment to the clavicle to expose the junction area between the internal jugular vein and the subclavian vein), and the dissection proceeds upwards along with the posterior surface of the SCM to expose the submandibular gland and the posterior belly of the digastric muscle. After flap dissection, the patient's head is returned to the neutral position. A spatula-shaped wide external retractor (Chung's retractor) is then used to raise and tent the skin flap at the anterior chest wall, the SCM, and the strap muscles to create a working space. The entire neck levels (level IIa, III, IV, Vb, and VI areas) are fully exposed by elevating the SCM muscle and the strap muscles. A second skin incision (0.8cm long) is then made on the medial side of the anterior chest wall to allow the fourth robotic arm to be inserted (2cm superiorly and 6-8cm medially from the nipple) (Fig. 5).

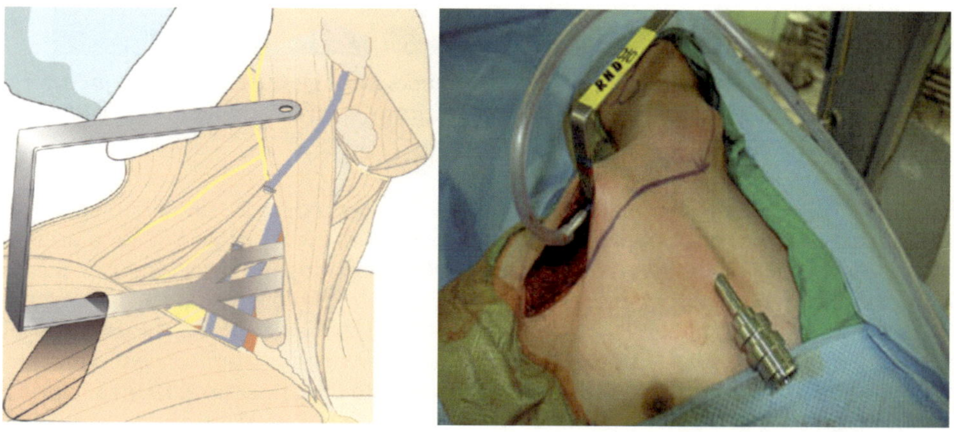

Fig. 5. Initial position of the external retractor during robotic modified radical neck dissection of levels III, IV, and Vb. The external retractor was placed between the thyroid and the strap muscle, with the direction of the blade from the axilla to the anterior neck (Kang et al, 2011).

2.6.2 Robot docking stage

The robotic column is placed on the lateral side of the patient contralateral to the main lesion, and the operative table is positioned slightly obliquely with respect to the direction of the robotic column to allow direct alignment between the axis of the robotic camera arm and the operative approach. Proper introduction angles are important to prevent collisions between robotic arms. Four robotic arms are used during the operation. Three arms are inserted through the axillary incision: a 30°degree dual channel camera is placed on the central camera arm through a 12-mm trocar. In particular, the camera arm should be placed in the center of the axillary skin incision. This arm is inserted to face upward. The 5-mm Maryland dissector is installed on the left side of the camera and the Harmonic curved shears on the right side through 8-mm trocar. A Prograsp forceps is placed on the fourth arm and inserted through the 8-mm anterior chest trocar. The Harmonic curved shear and the Maryland dissector arms should be inserted in the opposite manner to the camera arm (to face downward). Finally, the external three joints of the robotic arms should form an inverted triangle (Figure 6).

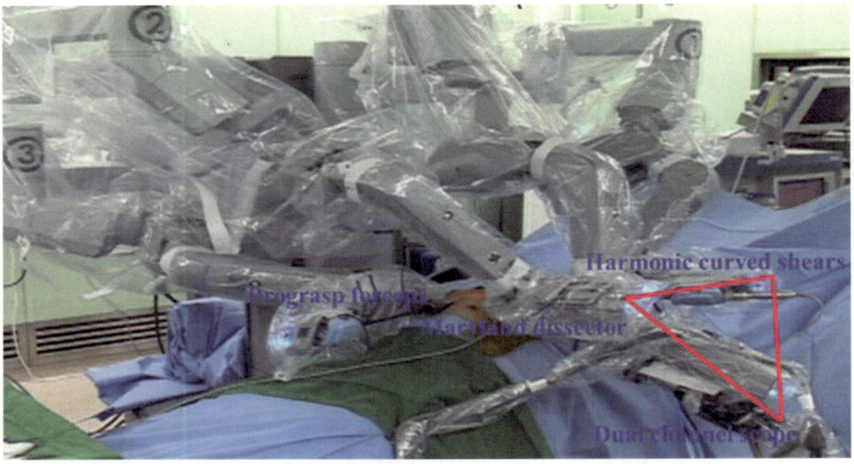

Fig. 6. Following the insertion of all robotic instruments through the axillary and anterior chest skin incisions, the three external joints of the robotic arms should form an inverted triangle.

2.6.3 Console stage

Actually, the robotic modified radical neck dissection procedure is similar to conventional open technique. Lateral neck dissection is initiated from the level III and IV area around the internal jugular vein (IJV). A careful dissection is needed during the detachment of the lymph node from the posterior aspect of the IJV to avoid injury to the common carotic artery and the vagus nerve. Smooth, sweeping, lateral movements of a Harmonic curved shears can establish a proper plane and allow vascular structures to be differentiated from specimen tissues. The dissection of the IJV is progressed upward from level IV to the upper level III area. During this procedure, the superior belly of the omohyoid muscle is cut at the thyroid cartilage level. Packets of LNs are then drawn superiorly using the ProGrasp forceps, and the LNs are meticulously detached from the junction of the IJV and subclavian vein.. In general, the transverse cervical artery courses laterally across the anterior scalene muscle, anterior to the phrenic nerve. Using this anatomic landmark, the phrenic nerve and transverse cervical artery can be preserved without injury or ligation. Further dissection is followed along the subclavian vein laterally. The inferior belly of omohyoid muscle is cut where it meets the trapezius muscle. The distal external jugular vein is then clipped and divided at its connection with the subclavian vein. Level VB dissection in the posterior neck area proceeds along the spinal accessory nerve in the superomedial direction, and is followed by level IV dissection, while preserving the brachial nerve plexus, the phrenic nerve, and the thoracic duct. The dissection proceeds by making turns at levels VB, IV, and III, and then by proceeding upward to the level IIA area. The individual nerves of the cervical plexus are sensory nerves, and when encountered during dissection they are sacrificed to ensure complete node dissection, while preserving the phrenic nerve and ansa cervicalis.

After performing the level III, IV and VB node dissection, re-docking is needed for a better operating view to dissect the level II lymph node. The external retractor is then reinserted through the axillary incision and directed toward the submandibular gland (Fig 7).

The operating table should also be repositioned more obliquely with respect to the direction of the robotic column to allow the same alignment between the axis of the robotic camera arm and the direction of retractor blade insertion. Drawing the specimen tissue inferolaterally, soft tissues and LNs are detached from the lateral border of the sternohyoid

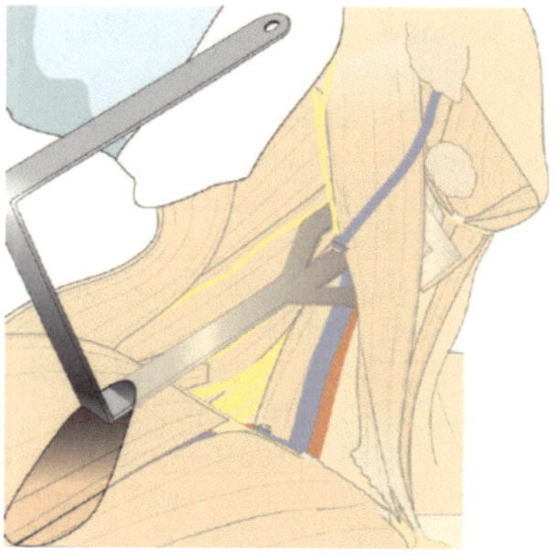

Fig. 7. Re-positioning of the external retractor during robotic modified radical neck dissection. For level II dissection, the blade of the external retractor is re-inserted toward the submandibular gland. (Kang et al, 2011).

muscle, the submandibular gland, and the anterior surfaces of the carotid artery and the IJV. Level IIA dissection is advanced until the posterior belly of the digastric muscle is exposed superiorly. After removing the specimen, fibrin glue is sprayed around the area of the thoracic duct and minor lymphatics, and a 3-mm closed suction drain is inserted just under the axillary skin incision. Wounds are closed cosmetically. The incision scar in the axilla is completely covered when the arm is in its neutral position.

3. Conclusion

A long journey has been traversed from the initial studies of lymphatic drainage of the neck, to determination of effective surgical extent and the development of effective surgical techniques for managing cervical nodal metastases in patients with head and neck cancers. Various neck dissection techniques have been utilized as a fundamental tool in the management of patients with head and neck cancer. The recently developed advanced robotic technique in head and neck surgery has been shown to be both safe and feasible in selected patients, yielding excellent cosmetic outcomes. Moreover, this technique may facilitate radical neck dissection during surgery for thyroid cancer. However, use of a robot for neck dissection of patients with head-and-neck cancer remains at an early stage, and prospective randomized studies are required to evaluate the real benefits afforded by this technique.

4. Acknowledgment

All authors including Drs. Lee, and Chung have no conflicts of interest or financial ties to disclose.

5. References

Bellantone, R.; Lombardi, CP. & Raffaelli, M. (2002) Central neck lymph node removal during minimally invasive video-assisted thyroidectomy for thyroid carcinoma: a feasible and safe procedure. *J Laproendosc Adv Surg Tech A*, Vol.12, No.3, pp. 181-185

Chung, WY. (2011) The evolution of robotic thyroidectomy: from inception to neck dissection. *J Robotic Surg*, Vol.5 pp.17-23

Dulquerov, P.; Leuchter, I. & Szalay-Quinodoz, I. (2001) Endoscopic neck dissection in human cadavers. *Laryngoscope,* Vol.111, No.12, pp.2135-2139

Dutta, S.; Slater, B, & Butler M. (2008) "Stealth surgery": transaxillary subcutaneous endoscopic excision of benign neck lesions. J Pediatr Surg, Vol.43, No.11, pp.2070-2074

Ferlito, A.; Rinaldo, A. & Siver, CE. (2006) Neck dissection: then and now. *Auris Nasus Larynx,* Vol.33, No.4, pp.365-374

Ferlito, A.; Siver, CE. & Rinaldo, A. (2008) Neck dissection: present and future? *Eur Arch Otorhinolaryngol,* Vol.265, No.6, pp.621-626

Ferlito, A; Robbins, KT. & Silver, CE. (2009) Classification of neck dissections: an evolving sytem. *Auris Nasus Larynx,* Vol.36, No.2, pp.127-134

Kang, SW.; Lee, SH. & Ryu, HR. (2010) Initial experience with robot-assisted modified radical neck dissection for the management of thyroid carcinoma with lateral neck node metastasis. *Surgery,* Vol.148, No.6, pp.1214-1221

Kazi, RA. (2003) The life and times of George Washinton Crile. *J Postgrad Med,* Vol.49, pp.289-290

Kitagawa, W.; Shimizu, K. & Akasu, H. (2003) Endoscopic neck surgery with lymph node dissection for papillary carcinoma of the thyroid using a totally gasless anterior neck skin lifting method, *J Am Coll Surg,* Vol.196, No.6, pp.990-994

Kowalski, LP. & Sanabria, A. (2007) Elective neck dissection in oral carcinoma: a critical review of the evidence. *Acta Otorhinolaryngol Ital,* Vol.27, No.3, pp.113-117

Lombardi, CP.; Raffaelli, M. & Princi, P. (2007) Minimally invasive video-assisted functional lateral neck dissection for metastatic papillary thyroid carcinoma. *Am J Surg,* Vol.193, No.1, pp. 114-118

Martin, H; Del Valle, B. & Ehrlich, H. (1951) Neck dissection. *Cancer,* Vol.4, No.3, pp.441-499

Miccoli, P. & Materazzi G. (2004) Update on endoscopic cervical surgery. *Semin Laparosc Surg,* Vol.11, No.3, pp.139-145

Muenscher, A.; Dalchow, C. & Kutta, H. (2011) The endoscopic approach to the neck: a review of the literature, and overview of the various techniques. *Surg Endosc,* Vol.25, No.5, pp.1358-1363

Richtsmeier, WJ. (2003) Dissecting the "endoscopic neck". *Arch Otolaryngol Head Neck Surg,* Vol.129, No.6, pp.612

Rinaldo, A.; Ferlito, A. & Silver, CE. (2008) Early history of neck dissection. *Eur Arch Otorhinolaryngol,* Vol.265, No.12, pp.1535-1538

Robbins, KT.; Clayman, G. & Levine, PA. (2002) Neck dissection classification update: revisions proposed by the American Head and Neck Society and the American Academy of Otolaryngology-Head and Neck Surgery. *Arch Otolaryngol Head neck Surg,* Vol.128, No.7, pp.751-758

Robbins, KT; Shaha, AR. & Medina, JE. (2008) Consensus statement on the classification and terminology of neck dissection. *Arch Otolaryngol Head Neck Surg,* Vol.134, No.5, pp.536-538

Seethala, RR. (2009) Current state of neck dissection in the United States. *Am J Surg Pathol,* Vol.34, No.8, pp.1106-1121

Terris, DJ.; Monfared, A. & Thomas, A. (2003) Endoscopic selective neck dissection in a porcine model. *Arch Otolaryngol Head Neck Surg,* Vol.129, No.6, pp.613-617

Ward, GE. & Robben, JO. (1951) A composite operation for radical neck dissection and removal of cancer of the mouth. *Cancer,* Vol.4, No.1, pp.98-109

Werner, JA.; Sapundzhiev, NR. & Teymoortash, A. (2004) Endoscopic sentinel lymphadenectomy as a new diagnostic approach in the N0 neck. *Eur Arch Otorhinolaryngol,* Vol.261, No.9, pp.463-468

7

Surgical Management of the Spinal Nerve in Modified Radical Neck Dissection

Attilio Carlo Salgarelli and Pierantonio Bellini
Unit of Maxillofacial Surgery
Head and Neck Surgery Department
University of Modena and Reggio Emilia
Italy

1. Introduction

In 1906, Crile (1906) first reported radical neck dissection as a surgical technique for the treatment of neck lymph-node metastasis of head and neck cancer. It began to be used more widely after the report of Martin et al. (1951). The basic technique for neck dissection involves excising the neck lymphatic tissue, together with the accessory nerve, sternocleidomastoid muscle, and internal jugular vein, although this results in marked postoperative morphological and functional disorders. In particular, severing the accessory nerve is associated with postoperative shoulder dysfunction.

Various techniques for functional (conservative) neck dissection have been introduced to prevent such dysfunction, and these techniques have been modified in various ways (Bocca & Pignataro, 1967; Bocca et al., 1980; Eisele et al., 1991; Medina & Lorè, 2005; Suarez, 1963).

The original approach to functional neck dissection was reported by Osvaldo Suarez in 1963. Unlike radical neck dissection, functional neck dissection can prevent postoperative morphological and functional disorders by preserving the accessory nerve, sternocleidomastoid muscle, and internal jugular vein.

Over the past 40 years, there has been ongoing development of various nerve-, vein-, and muscle-preserving techniques. The most recent development is selective neck dissection, based on site-specific lymph drainage patterns. These conservative procedures have attempted to alleviate neck and shoulder morbidity and to ensure that oncological safety is not compromised (Bocca & Pignataro, 1967; Bocca, 1975; Bocca et al., 1980; Eisele et al., 1991; Medina & Lorè, 2005; Suarez, 1963).

Damage to the spinal accessory nerve generally leads to the condition known as "sloping shoulder syndrome" (Salgarelli et al., 2009), which consists of:

- numbness over the angle of the jaw and around the ear due to the associated injury to the transverse cervical and great auricular nerves;
- paralysis of the trapezius muscle, resulting in shoulder droop and difficulty in shoulder movement, especially abduction, although some patients retain almost full movement;
- pain, often the worst consequence of injury, resulting from traction of the unsupported shoulder on the brachial plexus or even a sensory element in the spinal accessory nerve;
- winging of the scapula, which occurs because trapezius paralysis allows the medial border of the scapula to lift off the chest wall.

Shoulder and neck pain associated with neck dissection are well recognized and are closely related to the quality of life of patients undergoing surgical treatment for head and neck cancer. Shoulder pain and dysfunction have been reduced using modified radical neck dissection that preserves cranial nerve XI. Radical neck dissection has been reported to cause greater pain and shoulder dysfunction than conservative procedures.

2. Anatomy

The spinal root of the accessory nerve arises from a column of motor neurons called the spinal nucleus, located in the lateral part of the grey matter of the cervical region of the spinal cord. Its filaments arise from segments C1–C6 and emerge to form a trunk, then ascend through the foramen magnum with the vagus nerve to enter the posterior fossa. They join briefly with the cranial root, whose origins lie in the posterolateral groove of the medulla, to form a single trunk, which leaves the base of the skull via the jugular foramen to reach the retrostyloid space. The common trunk terminates here in the cranial and spinal roots, the former joining the superior ganglion of the vagus nerve and the latter passing obliquely downward and laterally either anterior or posterior to the internal jugular vein, or rarely through it. The point where the nerve crosses the jugular vein can be identified by locating the transverse process of the atlas.

Comparative anatomic studies show that the cranial nerve root connections of the spinal accessory nerve are variable, and may be intra- or extracranial (Kaji et al., 2001; Symes & Ellis, 2005; Younossi-Hartenstein et al., 2001). This can result in differing composition of the nerve, which may in part explain why different impairments can occur in different patients when nerves in the same location are cut. Variation has been documented in both the course of the nerve in the posterior triangle and in its distribution and branches (Caliot et al., 1989; Krause et al., 1991; Soo et al., 1986).

After crossing the internal jugular vein, the accessory nerve descends obliquely downward and backward to the upper part of the sternocleidomastoid muscle. It gives off a branch into the deep surface of this muscle and passes downward and backward, either deep to the sternocleidomastoid muscle or through it, to course across the posterior triangle. The nerve leaves the sternocleidomastoid muscle 0–3.8 (average 1.53) cm above Erb's point (Salgarelli et al., 2009).

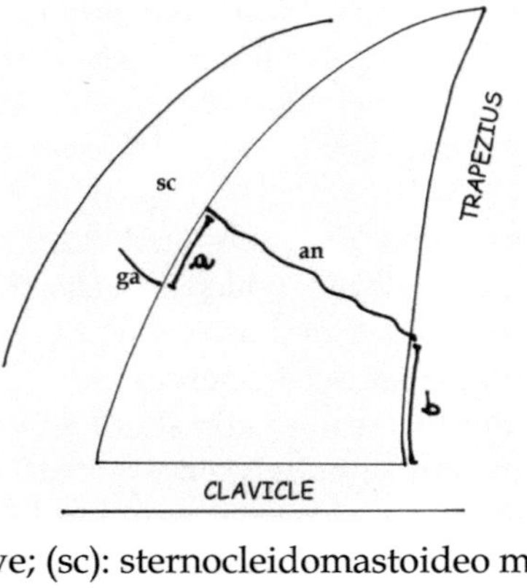

Fig. 1. (ga): great auricular nerve; (sc): sternocleidomastoideo muscle; (an): spinal accessory nerve; (a): distance between great auricular nerve and spinal nerve; (b): distance between clavicle and spinal nerve at the entrance of the trapezius muscle.

At Erb's point, the bundle of sensory nerves from the cervical plexus emerges from the posterior border of the sternocleidomastoid muscle (Aramrattana et al., 2005; Leung et al., 2004; Salgarelli et al., 2009), midway between the mastoid process and clavicle. Erb's point lies two finger-widths above the clavicle and one finger-width from the posterior border of the sternocleidomastoid muscle. At the great auricular point, the four branches (great auricular, lesser occipital, transverse cervical, and suprascapular) of the cervical plexus exit from the posterior border of the sternocleidomastoid muscle. In many surgical textbooks and in the recent literature, Erb's point has become synonymous with the great auricular point. In the posterior triangle, the nerve runs superficially, reaching the anterior border of the trapezius 2.5–7.3 (average 4.8) cm above the clavicle (Salgarelli et al., 2009).
Like the great auricular nerve, the spinal accessory nerve is often sandwiched tightly between the skin and muscle fascia, and the nerve can be injured when attempting to free up the skin in the lower lateral neck.

3. Identification of the spinal accessory nerve

From an oncological perspective, preservation of the spinal accessory nerve in modified neck dissections or lymph node biopsy is, when possible, the first objective in preserving shoulder function. To avoid iatrogenic injury, it is important to identify the course of the accessory spinal during the dissection.
The spinal accessory nerve must be identified as it enters the sternocleidomastoid muscle (anterior identification) if level 5 is not included in the neck dissection and at Erb's point (posterior identification) if level 5 is included in the neck dissection.

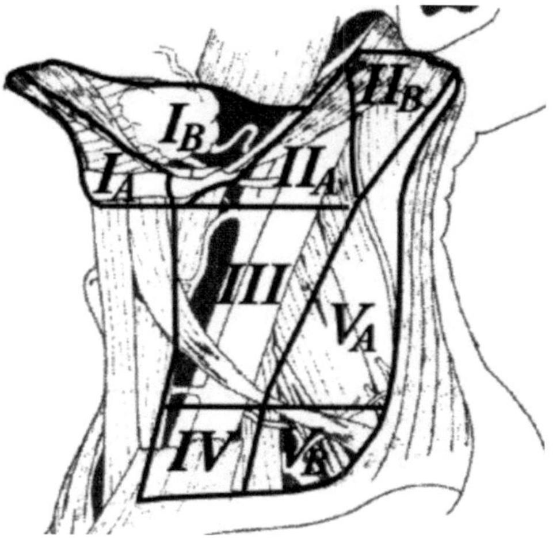

Fig. 2. Current limph node levels.
IA-submental limph nodes; IB-submandibular limph nodes; IIA-limph nodes located anterior to the vertical plane defined by the spinal accessory nerve; IIB- limph nodes located posterior to the vertical plane defined by the spinal accessory nerve; III-limph nodes located around the middle third of the internal jugular vein; IV-limph nodes located around the lower third of the internal jugular vein; VA-limph nodes located in the posterior triangle above the horizontal plane defined by the inferior border of the cricoid cartilage; VB- limph nodes located below the horizontal plane defined by the inferior border of the cricoid cartilage.

The literature describes myriad incisions for neck dissection (Bocca & Pignataro, 1967; Bocca et al., 1980; Holmes, 2008; Kademani & Dierks, 2005; Macfee, 1960; Medina & Lorè, 2005; Suarez, 1963). The choice of incision design in modified radical neck dissection is guided by the need to access the cervical lymphatic nodes at levels 1–5.

3.1 Anterior identification of the spinal accessory nerve

After the skin incision, a flap in the subplatysmal plain above the superficial layer of the deep cervical fascia is elevated to the level of the inferior border of the mandible.

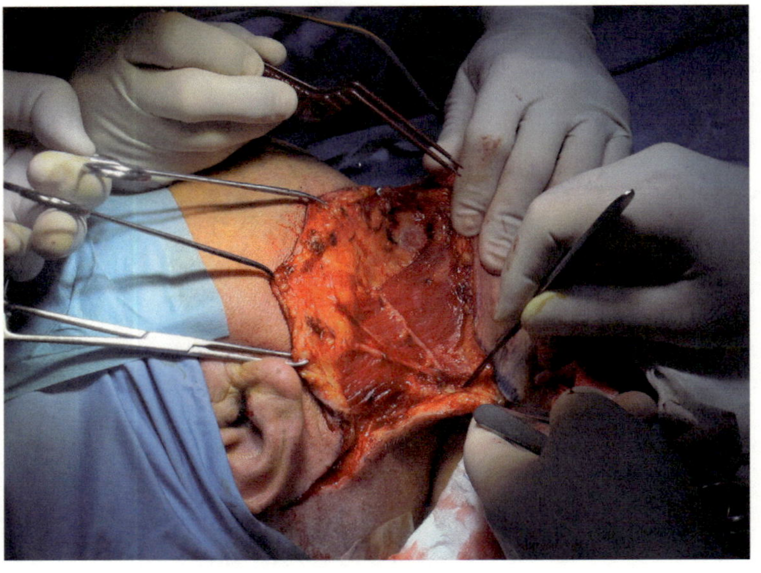

Fig. 3. Elevation of subplatismal flaps on the right side of the neck.

The external jugular vein serves as an excellent guide to keep this dissection at the appropriate level because the dissection should be superficial to it. An incision is then made through the fascia of the sternocleidomastoid muscle and this is elevated around the edge and onto the medial surface. The surgeon must be extremely careful in the upper half of this region, where the spinal accessory nerve enters the muscle. One or more small vessels usually accompany the spinal accessory nerve, which often divides before entering the muscle. The vessels should be cauterized without injuring the nerve, and all branches of the nerve must be preserved to obtain the best shoulder function.

After all of the small vessels entering the sternocleidomastoid muscle have been cauterized, the dissection continues posteriorly along the entire length of the muscle. The internal jugular vein can now be seen through the fascia of the carotid sheath. The dissection is carried upward to the level of the posterior belly of the digastric muscle.

The surgeon now moves to the upper part of the surgical field to complete the identification of the spinal accessory nerve; to approach this area, the sternocleidomastoid muscle is retracted posteriorly and the posterior belly of the digastric muscle is pulled superiorly with a smooth blade retractor, so the nerve is dissected toward the carotid sheath.

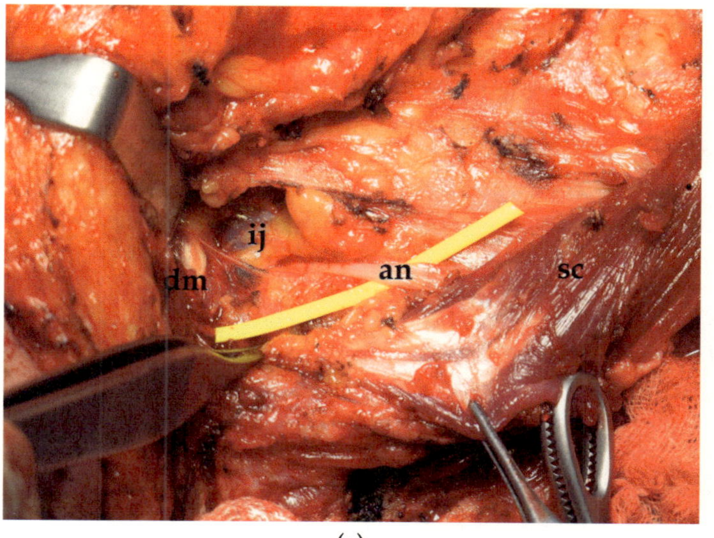

(a)

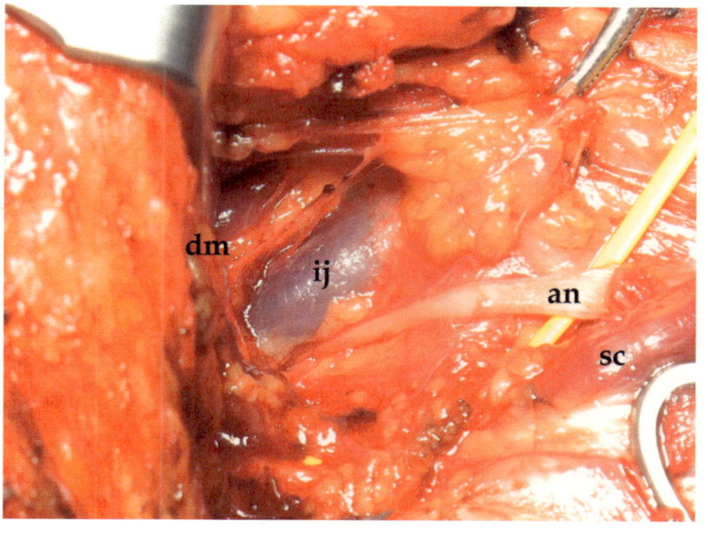

(b)

Fig. 4. Anterior identification of the spinal accessory nerve on the right side of the neck. (a) The spinal accessory nerve (an) is exposed (yellow landmark) between the sternocleidomastoid muscle (sc) and the internal jugular vein (ij). Posterior belly of digastric muscle (dm). (b) Closed view.

3.2 Spinal accessory nerve maneuver

The lymph nodes at level 2B are located between the spinal accessory nerve and internal jugular vein; this area has an ill-defined boundary and constitutes one of the weak points of the artificial lymph node classification. The surgeon must be especially careful during this step of the operation to avoid missing potentially metastatic lymph nodes.

At this level, the nerve runs within the "lymphatic container" of the neck, forcing the surgeon to cut across the fibro-fatty tissue. Consequently, the tissue overlying the nerve is divided and the nerve is exposed completely from the sternocleidomastoid muscle to the internal jugular vein. The nerve should be handled carefully, since manipulation alone can lead to long-term dysfunction.

As the dissection approaches the internal jugular vein, the surgeon must be aware of the relationship between these two structures. Usually, the internal jugular vein lies immediately behind the proximal portion of the nerve. On some occasions, however, the nerve may pass behind the vein or even across it.

Once the spinal accessory nerve has been exposed completely, the tissue lying superior and posterior to the nerve must be dissected from the splenius capitis and levator scapulae muscles. The tissue is pulled in an anteroinferior direction toward the spinal accessory nerve.

The deep cervical fascia overlying the splenius capitis and levator scapulae should be preserved. Care must be taken not to injure the internal jugular vein at this level, as control of the subsequent bleeding can be troublesome.

The occipital and sternocleidomastoid arteries are often found at this step of the operation. Most of the time, they are sectioned inadvertently while removing the lymphatic tissue in this area.

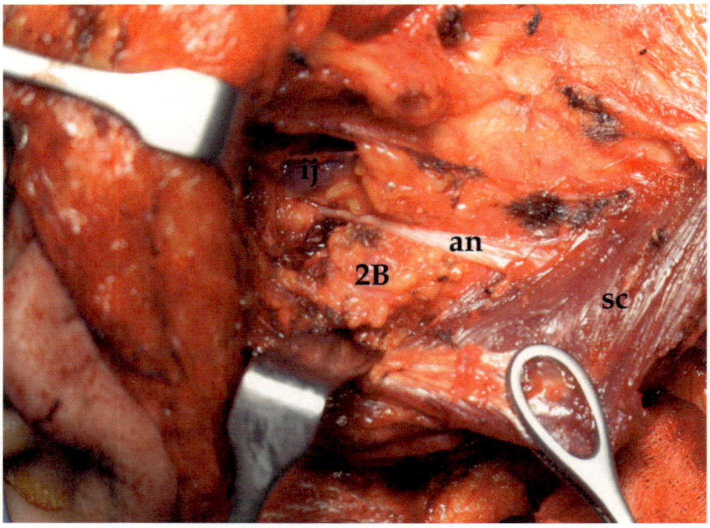

Fig. 5. Spinal accessory nerve maneuver on the right side of the neck. The fibrofatty tissue of the upper spinal accessory region has been dissected from the muscolar floor.

Then, fibro-fatty node-bearing tissue is passed under the spinal accessory nerve and kept in continuity with the reminder of the neck dissection. Osvaldo Suarez referred to this step of the operation as "the spinal accessory maneuver" (Suarez, 1963).

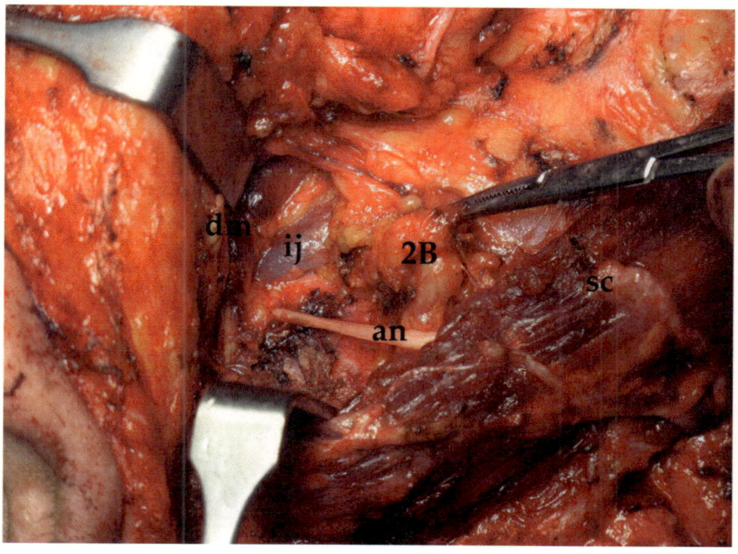

Fig. 6. Spinal accessory nerve maneuver on the right side of the neck. Intraoperative image demonstrating passing node under spinal accessory nerve (an) following dissection level 2B. Note right angle retraction of posterior belly of digastric muscle (dm) and sternocleidomastoid muscle (sc). Internal jugular vein (ij).

Note that the lymph nodes that are now being removed are located between the spinal accessory nerve and internal jugular vein. This region corresponds to the ill-defined boundary between level 2 and the upper part of level 5. Therefore, the surgeon must be especially careful during this step of the operation to avoid missing potentially metastatic lymph nodes.

3.3 Posterior identification of the spinal accessory nerve

If level 5 is included in the neck dissection, the spinal accessory nerve must be identified at Erb's point. An inferior flap in the subplatysmal plain is elevated to the level of the clavicle. The platysma muscle terminates posteriorly, and in this area, the dissection will be in a subcutaneous plane. The spinal accessory nerve exits the posterior border of the sternocleidomastoid muscle in the posterior neck triangle an average of 1–1.5 cm from the great auricular nerve in a deeper layer above the investing deep fascia (Kazunari et al., 2007; Salgarelli et al., 2009). The spinal accessory nerve leaves the sternocleidomastoid muscle and descends obliquely downward and backward toward the trapezius muscle in a subcutaneous plane. Care must be taken to identify and protect the spinal accessory nerve when a flap is developed here.

Anatomical landmarks define the boundaries of the surgical field in the posterior triangle (level 5). The posterior margin is marked by the anterior edge of the trapezius muscle; the upper boundary is defined by the exit of the spinal accessory nerve toward the trapezius muscle. The inferior limit is located at the level of the clavicle; on the left side, the surgeon must be aware of the variable anatomy of the thoracic duct when approaching the junction of the internal jugular and subclavian veins (levels 4 and 5). The transverse cervical vessels and omohyoid muscle constitute important anatomical landmarks within this area.

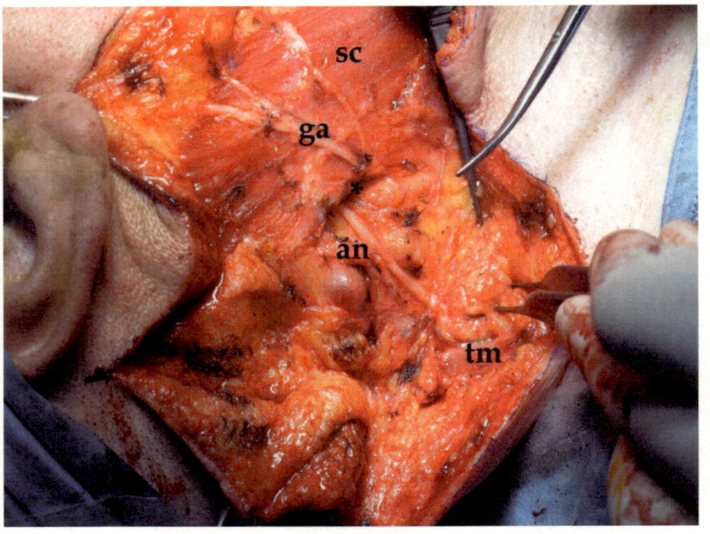

(a)

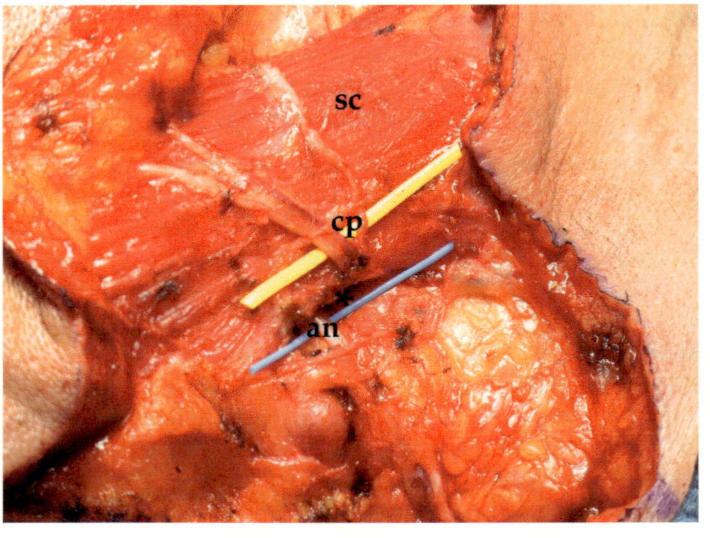

(b)

Fig. 7. Posterior identification of the spinal accessory nerve on the right side of the neck. (a) The spinal accessory nerve (an) is identified as it enters the sternocleidomastoid muscle (sc), usually at the junction of the upper third and lower two thirds of the muscle. Note the Erb's point (*) and the relations between spinal accessory nerve and the branches of the cervical plexus (great auricular nerve: ga). Trapezius muscle (tm). (b) Closed view: blue landmark on spinal accessory nerve (an) and yellow landmark on cervical plexus (cp).

The operation proceeds while keeping the spinal accessory nerve in view with the removal of the fascia that still covers the posterior border of the sternocleidomastoid muscle. Once completed, this maneuver results in the total release of the muscle from its surrounding fascia.

Then, the dissection proceeds from the anterior border of the trapezius muscle in a medial direction, including the lymphatic contents of the supraclavicular fossa.

4. Conclusion

The preservation of the spinal accessory nerve is essential in neck dissection and guarantees function of the scapula and avoids "sloping shoulder syndrome". The spinal accessory nerve must always be identified at the junction of the upper third and middle third on the medial aspect of the sterocleidomastoid muscle (anterior identification); if the level 5 should be included in the dissection, the nerve must also be identified at Erb's point (posterior identification). Identifying the accessory nerve based on the great auricular nerve should be suitable during surgery, since the great auricular nerve lies in a deeper layer under the investing deep fascia and over the prevertebral fascia. Since the great auricular nerve represents a constantly identifiable landmark, it allows simple and reliable identification of the course of the spinal accessory nerve.

5. References

Aramrattana A, Sittitrai P, Harnsiriwattanagit K (2005) Surgical anatomy of the spinal accessory nerve in the posterior triangle of the neck. *Asian J Surg* 28: 171–3.

Bocca E, Pignataro O. (1967) A conservation technique in radical neck dissection. *Ann Oto Rhino Laryngol* 76: 975-8.

Bocca E, Pignataro O, Sasaki CT (1980) Functional neck dissection, a description of operative technique. *Arch Otolaryngol* 106: 524–7.

Bocca E. (1975) Conservative neck dissection. *Laryngoscope* 85: 1511-5.

Caliot PH, Cabaine P, Bousquet V, Midy D (1989) A contribution to the study of the accessory nerve: surgical implications. *Surg Radiol Anat* 11: 11-5.

Crile G (1906) Excision of cancer of head and neck. JAMA 47: 1780–6.

Eisele DW, Weymuller EA, Price JC (1991) Spinal accessory nerve preservation during neck dissection. *Laryngoscope* 101: 433–5.

Kademani D, Dierks EJ. (2005) A straight-line incision for neck dissection: technical note. *J Oralmaxillofac Surg* 63: 563-3.

Kaji T, Aizawa S, Uemura M, Yasuki K (2001) Establishment of the left right asymmetric innervation of the Lancelot oral region. *J Comp Neurol* 435: 394–405.

Kazunari S, Shinichi A, Hiroko A, Satoshi M, Koji S, Masatsugu H, Yoshinobu I. (2007) Anatomical study of accessory nerve innervation relating to functional neck dissection. *J Oral Maxillofac Surg* 65:22-29

Krause HR, Bremerich A, Hermann M (1991) The innervation of the trapezius muscle in connection with radical neck dissection— an anatomical study. *J Craniomaxillofac Surg* 19: 87–9.

Holmes JD. (2008) Neck dissection: nomenclature, classification and technique. *Oral Maxillofacial Surg Clin N Am* 20: 459-75.

Leung MKS, Dieu T, Cleland H (2004) Surgical approach to the accessory nerve in the posterior triangle of the neck. *Plast Rec Surg* 6: 2067–70.

Macfee WF. (1960) Transverse incisions for neck dissection. *Ann Surg* 151: 279–84.

Martin H, Del Valle B, Ehrlich H, Cahan WG (1951) Neck dissection. *Cancer* 4: 441–99.

Medina JE, Lorè JM. (2005) The neck, In: Lorè JM, Medina JE, *Anatomic atlas of head and neck surgery*, 804, Elsevier, Philadelphia.

Salgarelli AC, Landini B, Bellini P, Multinu A, Consolo U, Collini M. (2009) A simple method of identifying the spinal accessory nerve in modified radical neck dissection: anatomic study and clinical implications for resident training. *Oral Maxillofac Surg* 13: 69-72.

Soo KC, Guiloff RJ, Oh A, Della Rovere GQ, Westbury G (1986) Innervation of the trapezius muscle: a study in patients undergoing neck dissection. *Head Neck Surg* 12: 488–95.

Suarez O (1963) El problema de las metastasis linfaticas y alejadas del cacer de laringe e hipofargine. *Rev Otorhinolaryngol* 23: 83–9.

Symes A, Ellis H (2005) Variations in the surface anatomy of the spinal accessory nerve in the posterior triangle. *Surg Radiol Anat* 27: 404–8.

Younossi-Hartenstein A, Jones M, Hartenstein V (2001) Embryonic development of the nervous system of the temnocephalid flatworm Craspedella pedum. *J Comp Neurol* 435: 259–62.

8

Management for the N0 Neck of SCC in the Oral Cavity

Masaya Okura, Natsuko Yoshimura Sawai,
Satoshi Sumioka and Tomonao Aikawa
*The First Department of Oral and Maxillofacial Surgery,
Osaka University Graduate School of Dentistry,
Japan*

1. Introduction

The oral cavity is the most predominant location in the head and neck region for primary malignant tumors, and more than 90 % cancer consists of squamous cell carcinoma (SCC).(Shah and Patel 2003) SCC has a high propensity to early and extensive lymph node metastases. Regarding cancer stage distribution at diagnosis, regional spread is more frequent in cancers of oral cavity and pharynx compared to other cancers, including such as prostate, breast, lung and bronchus, and colorectum (Figure 1).(Jemal *et al.* 2010) Therefore, clinicians for cancers of the oral cavity and pharynx have to regard regional metastasis as most important. Advanced SCC of the oral cavity has regional metastasis frequently, and even in small tumors (T1 or T2) has a relatively high propensity of regional lymph node

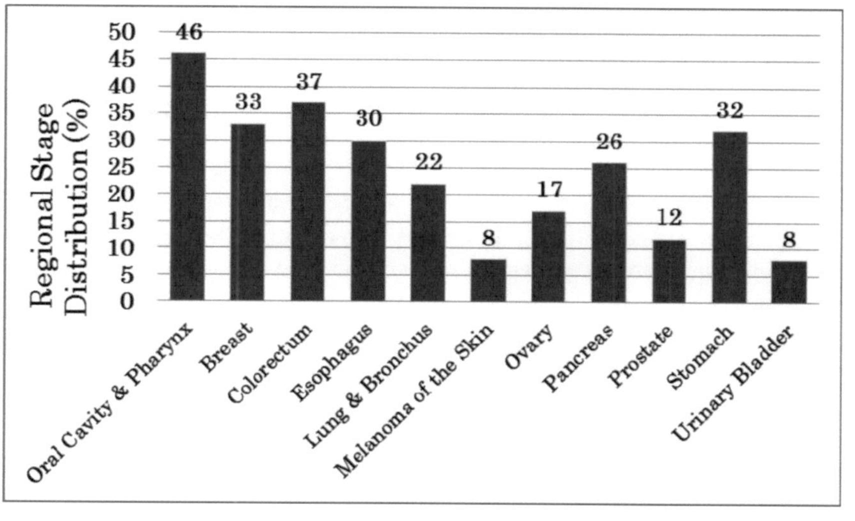

Fig. 1. Regional stage distribution of selected cancers, United States, 1999 to 2005.
Source: Horner M, Ries L, Krapcho M, et al, eds. SEER Cancer Statistics Review, 1975-2006. Bethesda, MD: National Cancer Institute; 2009.

metastasis. The five-year relative survival rate of patients who present with tumors localized at the primary site without dissemination to regional lymph nodes is 82%.(SEER, Oral cancer statistics, http://seer.cancer.gov/statfacts/html/oralcav.html) On the other hand, once dissemination to regional lymph nodes takes place, the survival rate reduces to nearly 50%. Advancement of regional disease, such as extracapsular spread and multiple nodal metastases, has influenced survival.(Myers *et al.* 2001; Shaw *et al.* 2009) Clearly, the regional status is the most significant independent prognostic factor,(Okura 2002; Shah *et al.* 1993; Taniguchi and Okura 2003) and appropriate management of the cervical lymph nodes is essential for control of disease.(Ferlito *et al.* 2006) In this chapter, we review the literature to ascertain whether elective neck dissection should be performed for cN0 neck or wait-and-see policy is safe and adequate.

1.1 Treatment of clinical N0 (cN0) neck

The management of neck disease in head and neck cancer, including oral cavity cancer, has been considered one of the most important aspects of treatment. When nodal metastases are present, nobody can deny the important effect of therapeutic neck dissection in the prognosis of head and neck cancer patients. However, the role of elective neck dissection has been a matter of discussion. Even the patients with clinically negative nodes (cN0) may still harbor occult metastasis, although advances in imaging techniques such as computed tomography, magnetic resonance, ultrasound sonography (US), and positron emission tomography have increased the accuracy of nodal metastases (Figure 2).

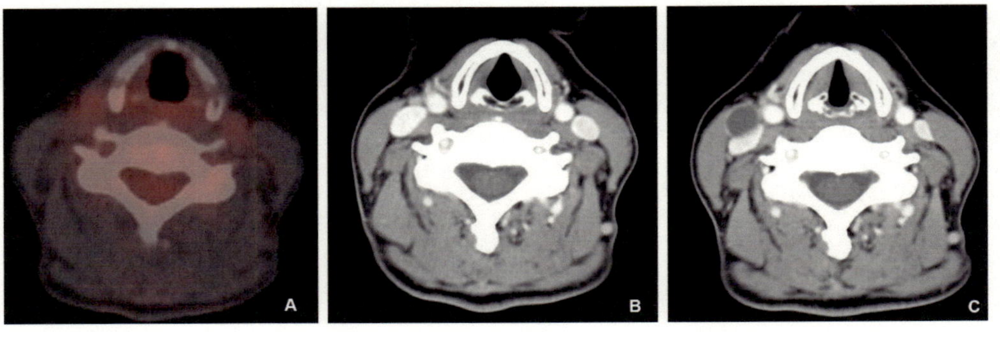

Fig. 2. Imagings of a patient with T2N0M0 SCC of the oral tongue.
A, preoperative positron emission tomography; B, preoperative enhanced computer tomography; C, enhanced computer tomography two months after transoral excision of the tumor. Preoperative assessment shows no involved node in the neck (A, B). Note late cervical nodal metastasis in the right side of the neck (Level III, C).

Table 1 shows the results of neck metastases and of each imaging study per patient with SCC of the oral tongue. CT had 70% accuracy, MRI had 74%, and US had 83% accuracy. Among the three image techniques US had the highest accuracy, although the accuracy was dependent on the observer. Our policy is essentially wait-and-see, and most of false-negative nodes were detected within 12 months after the initial transoral excision. In this study of oral tongue 66 (69%) patients with cN0 neck received intraoral excison alone, and 16 (17%) developed late lymph node metastases. The rate of occult metastases was 17% for SCC of the oral tongue and 21% for SCC of the oral cavity. Since the occult metastatic rate of head and neck cancer ranges from 17—50% (average, 28%) in the literature (Table 2), the optimal method of management of clinical N0 neck remains controversial.

	CT		MRI		US	
	-	+	-	+	-	+
Pathologically negative[1]	65	15	27	5	39	3
Pathologically positive						
Therapeutic neck dissection	2	24	1	16	1	12
Elective neck dissection	5	0	2	0	1	0
Regional recurrence	16	1	7	0	6	2
Loco-regional recurrence	4	0	2	0	2	0
Total	92	40	39	21	49	17
Sensitivity	52%		62%		67%	
Specificity	81%		84%		93%	
Positive predictive value	63%		76%		82%	
Negative predictive value	74%		73%		83%	
Accuracy	70%		74%		83%	

Table 1. Image accuracy of nodal positivity in patients with SCC of the oral tongue.
[1]Pathologically negative includes patients who performed intraoral excision alone with no regional recurrence; CT, computed tomography; MRI, magnetic resonance imaging; US, ultrasound sonography; -, negative; +, positive. Number indicates patient number.

The N0 neck can be treated electively or can be carefully observed (wait-and-see), and the decision can be made from each own clinical experience (Table 1). Randomized controlled trial (RCT) is desired to determine which is preferred, however RCT is not easy task. So far four RCTs of the small sample size had been performed. Vandenbrouck et al.(Vandenbrouck *et al.* 1980) demonstrated that the survival rates were similar between two treatment arms in 75 patients with oral cavity cancer, whereas Fakih et al.(Fakih *et al.* 1989) (n = 70) and Klingerman et al.(Kligerman *et al.* 1994) (n = 67) found that elective neck dissection had significant benefit for patients with tumor thickness of more than 4 mm. In 2009, Yuen et al.(Yuen *et al.* 2009) demonstrated that disease-free survival was quite similar between two arms in 71 patients with SCC of the oral tongue. Thus, these four RCTs failed to impact on clinicians due to the inconsistency and small number of cases studied. In 1994 Weiss et al.(Weiss *et al.* 1994) created a decision tree analysis and demonstrated that when the probability of occult cervical metastasis is more than 20%, the neck should be electively treated. Since then a large number of studies(Dias *et al.* 2001; Ferlito *et al.* 2006; Greenberg *et al.* 2003; Haddadin *et al.* 1999; O'brien *et al.* 2000; Sano and Myers 2007; Wei *et al.* 2006) supported their recommendation and preferred elective treatment for N0 neck,(Andersen *et al.* 1996; Bourgier *et al.* 2005; Brazilian 1998; Byers *et al.* 1998; Dias *et al.* 2001; Ferlito *et al.* 2006; Franceschi *et al.* 1993; Greenberg *et al.* 2003; Haddadin *et al.* 1999; Huang *et al.* 2008; Kaya *et al.* 2001; O'brien *et al.* 2000; Sano and Myers 2007; Wei *et al.* 2006; Yuen *et al.* 1997) because their occult metastatic rates were much higher than 20% (Table 2). Currently, the National Cancer Comprehensive Network's adopted practice guidelines have recommended elective neck dissection for clinical N0 cancer of the oral cavity, oropharynx, hypopharynx and supraglottic larynx. (NCCN, 2011) These guidelines apply to the performance of elective neck dissections as part of treatment of the primary tumor.

Another reason of the preference for elective neck dissection is less morbidity of supraomoyhoid neck dissection (SOHND) compared to classical radical neck dissection.(Spiro *et al.* 1996) For primary tumors in the oral cavity the regional lymph nodes at highest risk for early dissemination by metastatic cancer are limited to Levels I, II, and III

Author, year	Primary site	T stage	Patient number	% of occult metastasis	Neck treatment
Ho, 1992	OT	T1-2	28	42	obs
Lim, 2004	OT	T1-2	56	32	obs
Goto, 2005	OT	T1-2	88	26	obs, END
Lim, 2006	OT	T1-2	54	28	obs, SOHND
Keski-Säntti, 2006	OT	T1-2	80	30	obs, END
Kligerman, 1994	OC	T1-2	67	43	obs, SOHND
Brazilian H&N, 1998	OC	T2-4	148	28	mRND, SOHND
Kaneko, 2002	OC	T1-4	868	17	obs, END
Amaral, 2004	OC	T1-2	117	23	END
Smith, 2004	OC	T1-2	150	28	obs, END
Zbären, 2006	OC	T1-3	100	20	SOHND
Clark, 2006	OC	T1-4	105	34	obs, END
Mathew lype, 2008	OC	T1-4	219	27	SOHND
Okura, 2009	OC	T1-4	165	21	obs, END
Kraus, 1996	OC, OP	T1-4	44	32	SOHND
Nieuwenhuis, 2001	OC, OP	T1-2	161	21	obs
Duvvuri, 2004	OC, OP	T1-2	359	25	obs, END
O'Brien, 2008	OC, OP	T1-4	108	30	END
Spiro, 1996	H&N	-	268	25	SOHND
van den Brekel, 1999	H&N	T1-4	77	18	obs
Coatesworth, 2002	H&N	T1-4	63	30	END
Gourin, 2008	H&N	T1-4	337	50	END
Total			3662	28	

Table 2. Analysis of occult metastasis.
OT, oral tongue; OC, oral cavity; OP, oropharynx; H&N, head and neck; obs, observation; END, elective neck dissection; SOHND, supraomohyoid neck dissection; mRND, modified radical neck dissection.

in the supraomohyoid triangle. Skip metastasis to Levels IV and V in the absence of metastatic disease at Levels I, II, or III is exceedingly rare.(Shah *et al.* 1993) Compared to radical neck dissection SOHND reduces morbidity, including spinal accessory nerve disorder which results in diminished or absent function of the sternocleidomastoid muscle and upper portion of the trapezius muscle, and reduces cosmetic deformity. In addition, SOHND is considered as effective as comprehensive procedures for staging the clinically negative neck, when the neck is treated electively. It is intrinsic in the philosophy of a preventive treatment, to make it the less morbidity possible without losing oncologic results. However, this elective policy results in overtreatment of the neck, when the neck actually has no involved nodes. The less shoulder morbidity accompanied with SOHND is nonzero. Approximately 20% of patients who received SOHND had a shoulder pain even with conserving the accessary nerve.(Van Wilgen *et al.* 2004) Such overtreatment should be avoided when patients have no involved nodes in the neck.

1.2 Decision tree analysis

Upon returning decision tree analysis of Weiss et al., the decision tree is based on an analysis of the utility of the management options taking into account the incidence of node involvement, complications of treatment, and disease control rates.(Weiss *et al.* 1994) In sensitivity analysis they defined the expected utility to a function of the occult metastatic rate. They concluded that cN0 necks should be treated electively when the occult metastatic rate is more than 20%. The 20% of threshold has likely exerted a great influence on the management of cN0 necks, because they estimated curable probabilities using data of reviews published in the 1980s. Weiss et al. have however alluded that the values will change and the threshold will be altered with the times. The recommendation for elective neck dissection in more than two decades has to be reconsidered with the current data. Accordingly we have reconfigured the decision tree sensitivity analysis with our current disease control rates to determine optimal therapy based on a current set of underlying assumptions.(Okura *et al.* 2009) Two decision tree strategies for the management of cN0 neck was compared; elective neck dissection or wait-and-see. In sensitivity analysis the expected utility for each strategy is a function of occult metastatic rate according to Weiss study. The higher utility value is preferable to the lower one, and the intersection indicates the treatment threshold.

1.3 Formula of the threshold for the treatment of cN0 neck

The treatment threshold between elective neck dissection and observation was estimated with three (a–c) probabilities of survival; a = the curable probability (5-year overall survival rate) of the patients received elective neck dissection with no neck recurrence, b = the curable probability of the observed patients with late neck metastasis, c = the curable probability of the observed patients with no neck recurrence. These three probabilities are different in each institution. With the sensitivity analysis, the treatment threshold (Rx) can be calculated through the following:

$$\text{Rx} = (c - 0.97a)/(0.00376 - 0.0776a - 0.94b + c).$$

When clinicians calculate their own 3 probabilities (a–c) of being cured, they can estimate their own threshold for treatment of cN0 neck using this formula. The formula will be put to practical use and will estimate the current threshold. Our calculated threshold of the occult rate between the two strategies was 44.4% (Table 3). In our practice a patient with SCC of the oral cavity and N0 neck should be carefully observed if the probability of occult cervical metastasis is less than 44.4%. Only if the probability is greater than 44.4%, elective neck dissection might be warranted. Since the probability c is the survival rate for patients with no involved nodes who do not have occult metastases, c is expected to be a high rate. The probability a is the survival rate for patients who received elective neck dissection and should be lower than c, because some have occult metastases. If the occult metastatic rate is 0%, then the probability a would be quite same to c. A high occult metastatic rate and poor survival for patients with occult metastases contribute to a difference in probability between a and c.

Table 3 shows the treatment threshold in various three probabilities according to the formula. For instance, assuming that c is fixed to 80% and a is 65% gives Rx more than 30% when b is not less than 20%. Rx becomes greater in proportion to the increase of b, because the denominator in the formula is decreased. Assuming that a is 70%, Rx is more than 22%. Assuming that the difference between a and c is 5% (a = 75%), Rx is 13% when b = 20% and 16% when b = 30%, respectively. These Rx rates are too lower, however Rx goes up to more than 30% when b is more than 54%. Furthermore, providing that the difference between a and c is decreased to 2%, Rx is below 20% when b is less than 50%. For giving Rx > 30%, b needs more than 64%. It is therefore necessary for giving Rx high percentage to build up high *b* probability as well as the positive difference between *a* and *c*. First, we have to raise the successful salvage rate for patients with late neck metastases. In Table 3 when b is more than 60%, Rx is invariably over 24%.

a	*b*	*c*	Rx	
60%	50%	60%	21%	Weiss et al.
87.8%	71.3%	94.5%	44.4%	Okura et al.
65%	20%	80%	30%	
65%	30%	80%	36%	
70%	20%	80%	22%	
70%	30%	80%	26%	
70%	40%	80%	32%	
70%	50%	80%	43%	
75%	20%	80%	13%	
75%	30%	80%	16%	
75%	40%	80%	20%	
75%	54%	80%	30%	
75%	60%	80%	40%	
78%	30%	80%	9%	
78%	40%	80%	12%	
78%	50%	80%	16%	
78%	60%	80%	24%	
78%	64%	80%	31%	
78%	70%	80%	51%	

Table 3. Three probabilities (*a*–*c*) and treatment threshold (Rx).
Rx of our study (2009) was two times or more as high as that of Weiss study (1994). Rx is calculated with each *a, b* and *c* using the formula.

1.4 Predictors of occult metastases

The management of cN0 neck of SCC of the oral cavity is not necessarily wait-and-see (observation). In our study the overall occult rate was 21%, relatively low compared to other studies (Table 2) and our policy is wait-and-see. Notwithstanding, one-fifth of patients with cN0 neck need late neck dissection when all necks of those patients were observed. Patients with higher probability of occult metastases are encouraged to be selected with other predictors. For instance, our occult metastatic rate was 14% for T1 lesions, 23% for T2 lesions, and 30% for T3 lesions, respectively (Table 4).

T stage	Incidence	Rate
T1	21/152	14%
T2	54/232	23%
T3	16/53	30%
T4	7/38	18%
Total	98/475	21%

Table 4. Incidence and rate of occult metastases according to T stage.

The rate is increased in proportion of the increase of T stage, except for T4. The increase of primary lesions compels us to consider elective treatment, although the highest rate for T3 is still lower than our treatment threshold (44.4%). Other predictors of occult metastases are essential to management of cN0 necks.

Numerous studies have reported that histologic tumor thickness correlates closely with lymph node metastases in SCC of the oral cavity.(Asakage *et al.* 1998; Byers *et al.* 1998; Fukano *et al.* 1997; Lim *et al.* 2004; O-Charoenrat *et al.* 2003; Spiro *et al.* 1986; Yamazaki *et al.* 2004; Yuen *et al.* 2000) Patients with more than 3 - 6 mm of histologic tumor thickness recommends to treated electively because of high risk of metastases. However accurate preoperative assessment of the thickness in biopsy section is no easy task. It is occasionally difficult to reach an invasive front on biopsy, and the tumor thickness on biopsy is not necessarily the greatest. In order to detect tumor thickness more accurately, sequential sections are desirable but not pragmatic. Accordingly, multi-sliced imaging techniques should be useful and convenient.

Recently, the correlation between histologic tumor thickness and magnetic resonance imaging (MRI) tumor thickness was demonstrated (Iwai *et al.* 2002; Lam *et al.* 2004; Preda *et al.* 2006). Then MRI tumor thickness seems to become a candidate of occult metastatic predictor, although these studies did not reach to demonstrate the relation with MRI tumor thickness and regional metastases. We have verified MRI tumor thickness in patients with oral tongue SCC.(Okura *et al.* 2008) Coronal MRI was preferred to measure tumor thickness than axial image (Figure 3).

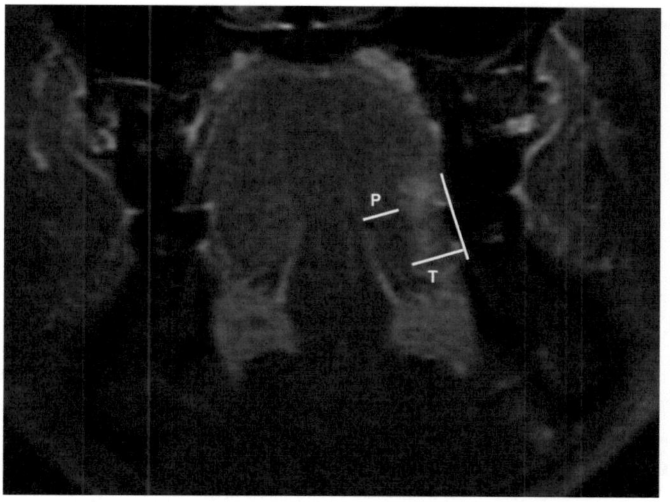

Fig. 3. Coronal contrasted-enhanced T1-weighted MRI shows tumor thickness (T) and paralingual distance (P). A vertical white line is a reference line connecting two tumor-mucosa junctions. A horizontal white line drawn perpendicular to the reference line represents radiologically is tumor thickness (T). The image shows that a high-intensity area, paralingual spatium, extends from the medial border of the sublingual space to the deep lingual artery along the genioglossus. The white line (P) is the paralingual distance between the tumor and the paralingual spatium.

Eighty-one % MRI permitted us the measurement of tumor thickness, however the remaining 19% could not be interpreted because of the interference of artifacts. There are some patients unsuitable for MR scan. Notwithstanding, MRI tumor thickness was related to lymph node metastases, and the mean of tumor thickness in patients with nodal metastases was twice length of that without nodal metastases. The thicker tumor thickness is, the higher the probability of lymph node metastases is (Table 5). Using logistic regression model, MRI tumor thickness was able to predict nodal metastasis in SCC of the oral tongue. Multivariate logistic regression function showed that if tumor thickness was 9.7mm, then the probalility of metastases was 20%. Tongue cancer varies in the growth pattern, endophytic or exophytic. Even if tumor thickness is similar in size, the position of the invasive front is different between endophytic and exophytic tumors. In order to observe where tumor cells invade, the paralingual distance between the invasive front and the paralingual spatium of tongue was measured (Figure 3). The paralingual spatium is loose connective tissue, which locates between the genioglossus muscle and the intrinsic tongue muscles to sublingual space. Lingual nerve and lingual artery run through this spatium, and the lingual artery is the landmark of this spatium. The paraligual distance was significantly related to lymph node metastases. The probability of nodal metastasis was in inverse proportion to the paralingual distance, and the probability was 20% at 5.2 mm of paralingual distance (Table 5). The two MRI parameters were more reliable than preoperative assessment of clinical N staging because of the log likelihood ratio. In our practice, when MR tumor thickness is more than 9.7 mm or paralingual distance is less than 5.2mm, we take elective neck dissection into consideration.

Probability of lymph node metastasis (%)	Tumor thickness (mm)	Paralingual distance (mm)
10%	7.1	6.5
20%	9.7	5.2
25%	10.6	4.7
30%	11.5	4.3
40%	12.9	3.6
50%	14.2	3.0

Table 5. Lymph node metastasis and measured MRI distances in SCC of the oral tongue.

Entering 5.2 mm of paralingual distance into the cut-off point resulted in 82% of specificity, 70% of sensitivity, and 14% of occult metastatic rate. The specificity of paralingual distance is higher than that using other images and the occult metastatic rate is the lowest (Table 1). Thus, MRI distances are useful to detect occult metastases of the oral tongue. Other endeavor to improve the accuracy of detecting occult metastases will be required.

2. Survival

In our study overall survival was similar, whether patients with cN0 neck are observed or electively treated. The 5-year overall survival rate for observed patients was 89%, and the rate for patients received elective neck dissection was 86% (Figure 4). On the other hand, patients with cN 1-3 neck had significantly lower overall survival (54% at 5-year) than those with cN0 neck.

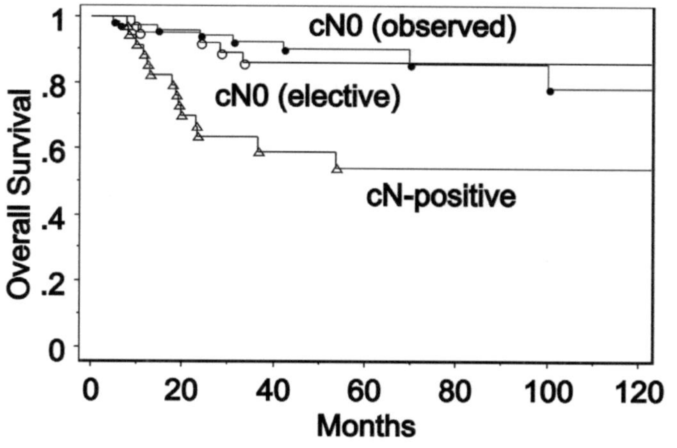

Fig. 4. Overall survival according to clinical N stage.
Clinical N0 necks were treated with two treatment arms: observation and elective neck dissection.

The outcome depends on the extent of the occult metastases at the time they are detected, which correlates with the intensity of follow-up.(Cheng and Schmidt 2008) In our practice, follow-up took place at every month in the first year, at two months in the second year, at three months in the third year, at four months in the fourth year, and 6 months in the fifth year. CT scan and ultrasound sonography were performed every half year. The follow-up is basic management, and the optional examinations are appended individually. For instance, patients with higher risk of lymph node metastases have ultrasound examination more times, and patients with higher risk of distant metastases have positron emission tomography test or pulmonary CT scan. It is important to understand which risks are high.

3. Conclusion

At present, it is impossible to set the incidence of occult metastases to zero. Additionally, more sensitive parameters or markers associated with the presence of nodal metastasis are encouraged to be developed. The continued advancement will have a significant impact on the evaluation, management and outcome of patients with the oral cavity. For the current management for the cN0 neck, the important points are: Clinicians have to comprehend their own threshold between observation and elective neck dissection. For that purpose, it is necessary to estimate the occult metastatic rate and three probabilities of survival (*a, b, c*). Then, the best policy of the management of cN0 necks is able to be controlled and determined.
Extended operations with less morbidity in surgical oncology have been pursued to improve the outcomes. However, these extended operations are not necessarily wise. Recently, extended para-aortic nodal dissection did not improve the survival of patients with gastric cancer,(Sasako *et al.* 2008) and axillary lymph node dissection should be considered unnecessary for woman with T1-2 invasive breast cancer.(Giuliano *et al.* 2011) Thus, some extended operations do not seem to be the standard treatment.
In SCC of the oral cavity, elective neck dissection does not also seem to be superior to a wait-and-see policy, and vice versa. Current studies, retrospective and prospective, have been unable to give us definitive recommendations regarding the management of the cN0

neck in those patients. However, the cN0 necks might be conserved more frequently without the decline of survival by means of the improvement of nodal assessment and the higher salvage rate of late lymph node metastases.

4. Acknowledgment

This work was conducted at the first department of Oral & Maxillofacial Surgery, Osaka University Dental Hospital in Japan. This work is supported in part by Grants from Ministry of Education, Science and Culture, Japan. We would like to express great gratitude to Chief professor Mikihiko Kogo and all clinical members in Osaka University Dental Hospital. We have furthermore to thank our secretary, Ms. Aya Okano to support this work.

5. References

Andersen, P. E., E. Cambronero, A. R. Shaha and J. P. Shah (1996) The extent of neck disease after regional failure during observation of the N0 neck. *Am J Surg* 172: 689-691, ISSN 0002-9610

Asakage, T., T. Yokose, K. Mukai, S. Tsugane, Y. Tsubono *et al.* (1998) Tumor thickness predicts cervical metastasis in patients with stage I/II carcinoma of the tongue. *Cancer* 82: 1443-1448, ISSN 1097-1042

Bourgier, C., B. Coche-Dequeant, C. Fournier, B. Castelain, B. Prevost *et al.* (2005) Exclusive low-dose-rate brachytherapy in 279 patients with T2N0 mobile tongue carcinoma. *Int J Radiat Oncol Biol Phys* 63: 434-440, ISSN 0360-3016

Brazilian, H., And, Neck, Cancer, Study, Group, (1998) Results of a prospective trial on elective modified radical classical versus supraomohyoid neck dissection in the management of oral squamous carcinoma. Brazilian Head and Neck Cancer Study Group. *Am J Surg* 176: 422-427, ISSN 0002-9610

Byers, R. M., A. K. El-Naggar, Y. Y. Lee, B. Rao, B. Fornage *et al.* (1998) Can we detect or predict the presence of occult nodal metastases in patients with squamous carcinoma of the oral tongue? *Head Neck* 20: 138-144, ISSN 1097-0347

Cheng, A., and B. L. Schmidt (2008) Management of the N0 neck in oral squamous cell carcinoma. *Oral and maxillofacial surgery clinics of North America* 20: 477-497, ISSN 1558-1365

Dias, F. L., J. Kligerman, G. Matos De Sa, R. A. Arcuri, E. Q. Freitas *et al.* (2001) Elective neck dissection versus observation in stage I squamous cell carcinomas of the tongue and floor of the mouth. *Otolaryngol Head Neck Surg* 125: 23-29, ISSN 0194-5998

Fakih, A. R., R. S. Rao, A. M. Borges and A. R. Patel (1989) Elective versus therapeutic neck dissection in early carcinoma of the oral tongue. *American journal of surgery* 158: 309-313, ISSN 0002-9610

Ferlito, A., A. Rinaldo, C. E. Silver, C. G. Gourin, J. P. Shah *et al.* (2006) Elective and therapeutic selective neck dissection. *Oral Oncol* 42: 14-25, ISSN 1368-8375

Franceschi, D., R. Gupta, R. H. Spiro and J. P. Shah (1993) Improved survival in the treatment of squamous carcinoma of the oral tongue. *Am J Surg* 166: 360-365, ISSN 0002-9610

Fukano, H., H. Matsuura, Y. Hasegawa and S. Nakamura (1997) Depth of invasion as a predictive factor for cervical lymph node metastasis in tongue carcinoma. *Head Neck* 19: 205-210, ISSN 1097-0347

Giuliano, A. E., K. K. Hunt, K. V. Ballman, P. D. Beitsch, P. W. Whitworth *et al.* (2011) Axillary dissection vs no axillary dissection in women with invasive breast cancer and sentinel node metastasis: a randomized clinical trial. *JAMA : the journal of the American Medical Association* 305: 569-575, ISSN 1538-3598

Greenberg, J. S., A. K. El Naggar, V. Mo, D. Roberts and J. N. Myers (2003) Disparity in pathologic and clinical lymph node staging in oral tongue carcinoma. Implication for therapeutic decision making. *Cancer* 98: 508-515, ISSN 1097-1042

Haddadin, K. J., D. S. Soutar, R. J. Oliver, M. H. Webster, A. G. Robertson *et al.* (1999) Improved survival for patients with clinically T1/T2, N0 tongue tumors undergoing a prophylactic neck dissection. *Head Neck* 21: 517-525, ISSN 1097-0347

Huang, S. F., C. J. Kang, C. Y. Lin, K. H. Fan, T. C. Yen *et al.* (2008) Neck treatment of patients with early stage oral tongue cancer: comparison between observation, supraomohyoid dissection, and extended dissection. *Cancer* 112: 1066-1075, ISSN 1097-1042

Iwai, H., R. Kyomoto, S. K. Ha-Kawa, S. Lee and T. Yamashita (2002) Magnetic resonance determination of tumor thickness as predictive factor of cervical metastasis in oral tongue carcinoma. *Laryngoscope* 112: 457-461, ISSN 1531-4995

Jemal, A., R. Siegel, J. Xu and E. Ward (2010) Cancer statistics, 2010. *CA: a cancer journal for clinicians* 60: 277-300, ISSN 1542-4863

Kaya, S., T. Yilmaz, B. Gursel, S. Sarac and L. Sennaroglu (2001) The value of elective neck dissection in treatment of cancer of the tongue. *Am J Otolaryngol* 22: 59-64, ISSN 0196-0709

Kligerman, J., R. A. Lima, J. R. Soares, L. Prado, F. L. Dias *et al.* (1994) Supraomohyoid neck dissection in the treatment of T1/T2 squamous cell carcinoma of oral cavity. *Am J Surg* 168: 391-394, ISSN 0002-9610

Lam, P., K. M. Au-Yeung, P. W. Cheng, W. I. Wei, A. P. Yuen *et al.* (2004) Correlating MRI and histologic tumor thickness in the assessment of oral tongue cancer. *AJR Am J Roentgenol* 182: 803-808, ISSN 0195-6108

Lim, S. C., S. Zhang, G. Ishii, Y. Endoh, K. Kodama *et al.* (2004) Predictive markers for late cervical metastasis in stage I and II invasive squamous cell carcinoma of the oral tongue. *Clin Cancer Res* 10: 166-172, ISSN 1557-3265

Myers, J. N., J. S. Greenberg, V. Mo and D. Roberts (2001) Extracapsular spread. A significant predictor of treatment failure in patients with squamous cell carcinoma of the tongue. *Cancer* 92: 3030-3036, ISSN 1097-1042

NCCN practice guidelines for cancer of the head and neck, version 2.2011, 05.08.2011, available from http://www.nccn.org/professionals/physician_gls/f_guidelines.asp

O'brien, C. J., S. J. Traynor, E. Mcneil, J. D. Mcmahon and J. M. Chaplin (2000) The use of clinical criteria alone in the management of the clinically negative neck among patients with squamous cell carcinoma of the oral cavity and oropharynx. *Arch Otolaryngol Head Neck Surg* 126: 360-365, ISSN 0886-4470

O-Charoenrat, P., G. Pillai, S. Patel, C. Fisher, D. Archer *et al.* (2003) Tumour thickness predicts cervical nodal metastases and survival in early oral tongue cancer. *Oral Oncol* 39: 386-390, ISSN 1368-8375

Okura, M. (2002) Lymph node metastasis. In: Pandalai SG, ed. *Rencent Research Developments in Cancer.* Vol 4. Part 1. Transworld Reseach Network, 331-337, ISBN 81-7895-051-0

Okura, M., T. Aikawa, N. Y. Sawai, S. Iida and M. Kogo (2009) Decision analysis and treatment threshold in a management for the N0 neck of the oral cavity carcinoma. *Oral Oncol* 45: 908-911, ISSN 1368-8375

Okura, M., S. Iida, T. Aikawa, T. Adachi, N. Yoshimura *et al.* (2008) Tumor thickness and paralingual distance of coronal MR imaging predicts cervical node metastases in oral tongue carcinoma. *AJNR Am J Neuroradiol* 29: 45-50, ISSN 0195-6108

Preda, L., F. Chiesa, L. Calabrese, A. Latronico, R. Bruschini *et al.* (2006) Relationship between histologic thickness of tongue carcinoma and thickness estimated from preoperative MRI. *Eur Radiol* 16: 2242-2248, ISSN 1432-1084

Sano, D., and J. N. Myers (2007) Metastasis of squamous cell carcinoma of the oral tongue. *Cancer Metastasis Rev* 26: 645-662, ISSN 1573-7233

Sasako, M., T. Sano, S. Yamamoto, Y. Kurokawa, A. Nashimoto *et al.* (2008) D2 lymphadenectomy alone or with para-aortic nodal dissection for gastric cancer. *The New England journal of medicine* 359: 453-462, ISSN 1533-4406

Shah, J. P., J. E. Medina, A. R. Shaha, S. P. Schantz and J. R. Marti (1993) Cervical lymph node metastasis. *Curr Probl Surg* 30: 1-335, ISSN 1535-6337

Shah, J. P., and S. G. Patel (2003) *Head and Neck Surgery and Oncology*. Mosby, London, ISBN 0-7234-3223-6

Shaw, R. J., D. Lowe, J. A. Woolgar, J. S. Brown, E. D. Vaughan *et al.* (2009) Extracapsular spread in oral squamous cell carcinoma. *Head Neck*, ISSN 1097-0347

Spiro, R. H., A. G. Huvos, G. Y. Wong, J. D. Spiro, C. A. Gnecco *et al.* (1986) Predictive value of tumor thickness in squamous carcinoma confined to the tongue and floor of the mouth. *Am J Surg* 152: 345-350, ISSN 0002-9610

Spiro, R. H., G. J. Morgan, E. W. Strong and J. P. Shah (1996) Supraomohyoid neck dissection. *Am J Surg* 172: 650-653, ISSN 0002-9610

Taniguchi, Y., and M. Okura (2003) Prognostic significance of perioperative blood transfusion in oral cavity squamous cell carcinoma. *Head Neck* 25: 931-936, ISSN 1097-0347

Van Wilgen, C. P., P. U. Dijkstra, B. F. Van Der Laan, J. T. Plukker and J. L. Roodenburg (2004) Shoulder and neck morbidity in quality of life after surgery for head and neck cancer. *Head & neck* 26: 839-844, ISSN 1043-3074

Vandenbrouck, C., H. Sancho-Garnier, D. Chassagne, D. Saravane, Y. Cachin *et al.* (1980) Elective versus therapeutic radical neck dissection in epidermoid carcinoma of the oral cavity: results of a randomized clinical trial. *Cancer* 46: 386-390, ISSN 0008-543X

Wei, W. I., A. Ferlito, A. Rinaldo, C. G. Gourin, J. Lowry *et al.* (2006) Management of the N0 neck--reference or preference. *Oral Oncol* 42: 115-122, ISSN 1368-8375

Weiss, M. H., L. B. Harrison and R. S. Isaacs (1994) Use of decision analysis in planning a management strategy for the stage N0 neck. *Arch Otolaryngol Head Neck Surg* 120: 699-702, ISSN 0886-4470

Yamazaki, H., T. Inoue, K. Yoshida, E. Tanaka, Y. Yoshioka *et al.* (2004) Lymph node metastasis of early oral tongue cancer after interstitial radiotherapy. *Int J Radiat Oncol Biol Phys* 58: 139-146, ISSN 0360-3016

Yuen, A. P., C. M. Ho, T. L. Chow, L. C. Tang, W. Y. Cheung *et al.* (2009) Prospective randomized study of selective neck dissection versus observation for N0 neck of early tongue carcinoma. *Head & neck* 31: 765-772, ISSN 1043-3074

Yuen, A. P., K. Y. Lam, W. I. Wei, C. M. Ho, T. L. Chow *et al.* (2000) A comparison of the prognostic significance of tumor diameter, length, width, thickness, area, volume, and clinicopathological features of oral tongue carcinoma. *Am J Surg* 180: 139-143, ISSN 0002-9610

Yuen, A. P., W. I. Wei, Y. M. Wong and K. C. Tang (1997) Elective neck dissection versus observation in the treatment of early oral tongue carcinoma. *Head Neck* 19: 583-588, ISSN 1043-3074

9

Neck Dissection of the Head and Neck Sarcoma

Yuki Saito and Takahiro Asakage
Department of Otolaryngology, Head and Neck Surgery,
The University of Tokyo,
Japan

1. Introduction

Sarcomas of the Head and Neck (SHN) are rare tumors of connective tissue origin that comprise less than 1% of head and neck malignancies. SHN account for approximately 5% to 10% of all sarcomas (Bruce, 2004). They arise in any soft tissue or osseous tissues of the region and may be found in patients of any age or gender. This chapter we will present the essential elements of diagnosis and resection or neck dissection of head and neck sarcoma.

Diagnosis of SHN is a diagnostic challenge. Although biopsy by FNA identified the correct specific sarcoma type in only 21% of cases, FNA led to an appropriate diagnostic biopsy in 88% (Costa et al., 1996). In only 7% of cases were the FNA findings misleading (benign or inflammatory) and in 5% of cases the reading was interpreted as inadequate. More recently, FNA biopsies of sarcoma were more often interpreted as showing a lower grade than that determined by final analysis of the fully resected specimen (Jones et al. 2002). Superficial and accessible lesions or lesions with inconclusive results from prior closed biopsy should be biopsied by incisional or excisional technique; fine needle aspiration or core needle biopsy should be reserved for deeper and less accessible lesions (Schalow & Broecker, 2003). Frequently the initial procedure for patients with a mass suspected to be Rabdomyosarcoma is a biopsy, usually open, which obtains an adequate specimen for pathological, biological and treatment protocol studies. There may be instances when core needle biopsy is appropriate, such as metastatic disease or small lesions in areas that will be treated primarily by chemotherapy and radiotherapy (Rodeberg et al, 2002). Since lymphoma and nasopharyngeal carcinoma would show the same signal intensity characteristics as sarcomas on magnetic resonance, tissue biopsy is imperative for correct diagnosis (Flympas et al. 2009).

The main therapy for soft tissue sarcomas of the head and neck is en-bloc resection with a margin of normal tissue. The adequacy of surgical resection seems to be a major determinant of outcome for sarcomas. The difficulty with en-bloc resection in these tumors relates to the proximity of important neurovascular structures and vital organs, as well as the cosmetic and functional morbidity resulting from such radical extirpative procedures. It is known that some soft-tissue sarcomas develop a pseudocapsule as a result of compression of adjacent tissues. This may obscure the true invasive nature of these neoplasms. Sarcomas tend to extend outside this pseudocapsule and invade tissues that may seem uninvolved during surgery. Because of the anatomical challenges of en-bloc resection for soft tissue sarcomas of the head and neck, positive margins should prompt the addition of adjuvant radiotherapy. Death from SHN is often a consequence of uncontrolled local disease as it is from metastases, unlike other sarcomas where local salvage options are often available.

Most soft tissue sarcoma spread in a longitudinal direction within the muscle groups where they originate. They generally respect barriers to tumor spread, such as bones, interosseous membrane, major fascial planes, etc, and this feature should be exploited in planning tissue preserving approaches to management. As they extend, lesions invade muscle and contiguous structures or other vital anatomy (de Bree et al, 2010).

Most SHN present with localized disease with metastasis being present in fewer than 10% of cases at the time of diagnosis and initial treatment. Predominant risk is to the lungs. Lymph node metastasis is considered an infrequent event in the natural history of soft tissue sarcomas. The rarity of such lymph node metastasis has made the study of their natural history difficult. Most published series are small, retrospective studies, and as individual studies are hard to interpret. The overall incidence of lymph node metastasis was estimated to be 10%. Lymphatic spread in sarcomas are rare, and that lymphatic spread is more frequently associated with certain histologic types. Those are, rhabdomyosarcomas, epithelioid sarcomas, angiosarcomas, and synovial sarcomas. Bone sarcomas may also present with regional lymph node disease, which carries a very adverse outcome. (Fong et al, 1993)

We discuss the previous reports of neck metastasis and neck dissection of main subtypes of Head and neck sarcoma.

1 Rabdomyosarcoma, 2 Fibrous tumor (desmoid tumor, fibrosarcoma, dermatofibrosarcoma protuberans), 3 Angiosarcoma 4 Synovial sarcoma, 5 Osteosarcoma, 6 Chondrosarcoma, 7 Ewing's sarcoma.

2. Rabdomyosarcoma

The rhabdomyosarcoma (RMS), a skeletal muscle subtype, is the most common soft tissue sarcoma in children, comprising about 50% of these tumors. In contrast, adult rhabdomyosarcomas comprise less than 10% of all soft tissue sarcomas. The head and neck are the most common primary sites for RMS in children and teenagers, followed by the genitourinary tract, limbs, thorax, and retroperitoneum. The tumor head and neck subsites include the orbit, parameningeal sites (nasopharynx, nasal cavity, paranasal sinuses, temporal bone, pterygopalatine fossa, and the infratemporal fossa), and non-parameningeal sites. Tumors that invade the orbit only have a better prognosis. (Moretti, 2010)

Subtypes may be histologically classified as: embryonic (which may be subdivided into embryonic, botryoid, and spindle cell tumors), alveolar, or pleomorphic. In children, about 60% are embryonic tumors, 20% are alveolar tumors, 15% are not classified, and 5% are pleomorphic tumors. The embryonic subtype has a better prognosis in children, but is more aggressive in adults. The alveolar subtype has a poor outcome because of its propensity to metastasize at a distance. The pleomorphic subtype occurs predominantly in adults. (World Health Organization Classification of Tumours [WHO] Tumors of Soft Tissue and Bone, 2010)

2.1 Treatment

Prior to the introduction of antineoplastic drugs, surgery played the central role in the cure of patients with RMS; in the last four decades, the development of multi-agent chemotherapy protocols resulted in a significant improvement in long-term survival: from 25% in 1970, to approximately 70% nowadays. In the head and neck area, a distinction is drawn between parameningeal rhabdomyosarcoma (PM-RMS) and RMS of other localizations. RM-RMS arises at sites with a particularly close anatomic relationship with the meninges such as nasopharynx, nasal cavity, paranasal sinuses, middle ear and mastoid, infratemporal and pterygopalatine fossa. They represent a particular surgical challenge. Surgical excision may lead to unacceptable mutilations and incomplete resection in most cases. These tumours have a high likelihood of meningeal extension, which is considered a fatal pattern of progression. Most authors conclude that multi-agent chemotherapy combined with radiation is the primary treatment modality offered to children with PM-RMS. Surgery prior to chemotherapy is recommended if there is no intracranial extension, if complete resection seems feasible and if it won't lead to unacceptable morbidity. (Gradoni, et al. 2010)

2.2 Lymphatic metastasis and neck dissection

Head and neck RMS has proven able to spread to cervical lymph nodes. Comparing the two most frequent histologic subtypes i.e. embryonal and alveolar, the latter showed a higher tendency to metastasize through the lymphatic route. According to some authors, elective treatment of the neck is not justified. In view of the low incidence of cervical lymph node metastases of merely 3% according to the IRS (Intergroup Rhabdomyosarcoma Study), Rodeberg et al. saw no indication for conducting elective neck dissection (Rodeberg et al.2002). Wurm recommends elective neck dissection in patients with alveolar RMS when surgery on primary tumour is planned (Wurm, 2005). Callender et al. found regional metastasis in 15–38% of their patients respectively and inferred that elective neck dissection offers a benefit (Callender, 1995). Controversy exists also over treating the N+ neck with additional radiotherapy or neck dissection. If nodes are metastatic and complete primary tumour resection is feasible, neck dissection is recommended; while, if the lymph nodes are positive but the primary tumour is unresectable, they should be included in the radiotherapy field.

2.3 Case report

An 22 year-old female, who had been treated for retinoblastoma at six months of age, presented for evaluation of left temporal swelling. She had underwent enucleation of the bilateral eyeball and 40 Gy irradiation to the left orbit at 1 years of age. Examination revealed a firm mass overlying the left temporal muscle (Figure 1) and left cervical

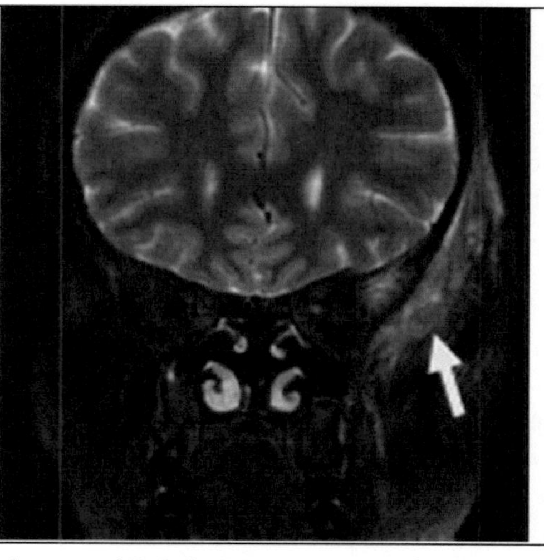

Fig. 1. A 22-year-old female case of Rabdomyosarcoma, infantile type of the temporal muscle (arrow). She underwent the convination of chemotherapy and radiation 9 years ago, now she was free of disease. (Our experience case)

lymphadenopathy. Biopsy revealed that the tumor was Rabdomyosarcoma, embryonal type. Metastatic work-up was negative including lumber puncture, bone scan ,and chest CT. The patient received treatment with chemotherapy consisting of vincristine 2 mg/m2 , actinomycin D 0.5 mg/m2,and cyclophosphamide 2.2g/m2 (VAC) every 3 weeks for 13 courses. Also she was irradiated 24Gy between 5 courses and 6 courses. She was followed closely after completing chemotherapy. The patient was alive and well with no evidence of disease 80 months after last treatment.

3. Fibrous tumor (Malignant fibrous histiocytoma, Desmoid tumor, and Fibrosarcaoma)

Since the late 1970s malignant fibrous histiocytoma (MFH) were the most common soft tissue sarcoma of middle and late adulthood. The existence of "malignant fibrous histiocytoma" as a distint entity is now considered controversial and at best is regarded ad a heterogeneous group of tumors without a specific known line of differentiation. Current nomenclature recognizes the entities undifferentiated high grade pleomorphic sarcoma, and myxofibrosarcoma (Montgomery et al. 2009).

Desmoid tumors, or aggressive deep-seated fibromatosis, are part of a rare group of fibrous tissue proliferations which tend to be locally aggressive but have no propensity for metastasis. Desmoid tumors are uncommon and slow-growing tumors with a propensity for recurrence even after complete resection. The natural history of desmoid tumors is not well-defined and poorly understood. Location of tumors can limit therapeutic options and result in significant morbidity with or without surgical resection. While there is no risk of degeneration from fibromatosis to fibrosarcoma, this is a distinct type of soft tissue sarcoma.Unfortunately, there are also no distinct clinical characteristics of fibrosarcoma, and disease is poorly described in the context of all fibroblastic tumors. Classic fibrosarcomas are seen in persons aged 30–55 years. Fibrosarcomas can be part of the spectrum of radiation-induced or radiation-associated sarcomas, representing about 15% of the histologic subtypes. Treatment options are dictated by location, and surgical resection remains the mainstay of curative therapy. Dermatofibrosarcoma protuberans (DFSP) is a specific form of soft tissue sarcoma which is nearly always considered a low-grade sarcoma. These tumors are prone to recurrence, with high local recurrence rates of up to 60% following resection. Occasionally, DFSP will undergo transformation to classic fibrosarcoma (Wong et al, 2008).

3.1 Treatment

The management of soft tissue sarcomas in the head and neck is primarily surgical. Sarcomas also tend to growth along fascial planes. For these reasons, the surgical resection of sarcomas require a wide resection which respects fascial compartments and includes a generous amount of uninvolved tissue beyond the tumour margins. For most cancer types, a 2.0- to 3.0-cm margin including resection of the underlying fascia is recommended. The critical anatomy of the head and neck limits the capacity to obtain these wide surgical margins. Sarcomas arising in the head and neck have a higher local recurrence rate and a worse disease-specific survival than sarcomas arising at other sites. (Brockstein, 2004)

3.2 Lymphatic metastasis and neck dissection

The incidence of lymph node metastasis of fibrosarcoma was found to be 4.4-5.1 %. It is generally agreed that because of the rarity of lymph node metastasis, elective neck dissection for fibrosarcoma is generally not indicated. (Fong et al, 1993)

3.3 Case report

A 62-year-old male was referred to our hospital for the left neck mass. He had been underwent the removal of the left neck mass and the pathological diagnosis was extra-abdominal desmoid. A MRI showed the high intensity mass of the Gd-enhanced T1 weighted image in the Level III area and infiltrate to the surrounding muscles (figure 2). He was underwent the removal of the tumor, encased by the sternocleidmastoid muscle and deep cervical muscles, with preservation of the internal juglar vein and phenic nerve. He was free of disease after the 3 years.

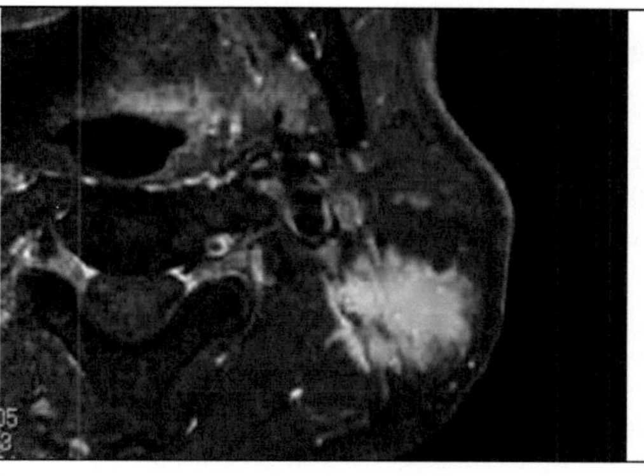

Fig. 2. A 62-year-old male case of desmoid. He underwent the removal encased by the surrounding muscles. After the 3 years operation, now he was free of disease. (Our experience case)

4. Angiosarcoma

Angiosarcomas are a subtype of soft-tissue sarcoma and are aggressive, malignant endothelial-cell tumors of vascular or lymphatic origin (Young et al, 2010). Treatment is challenging in many cases and the prognosis is poor. Angiosarcoma can arise in any soft-tissue structure or viscera and cutaneous angiosarcomas typically involve the head and neck, particularly the scalp (27%). Angiosarcomas are subdivided into cutaneous angiosarcoma, lymphoedema-associated angiosarcoma, radiation-induced angiosarcoma, rimary-breast angiosarcoma, and soft-tissue angiosarcoma, and most reports include several angiosarcoma subtypes. There is some evidence that tumor behaviour might depend on site of origin, although whether differences between cutaneous, radiation induced, breast, and visceral angiosarcomas are caused by biological differences or differences in clinical presentation and treatment is unclear.

4.1 Treatment

There are no randomised trials and few prospective studies, most published reports of angiosarcoma treatment are retrospective case series. Treatment has been included in management guidelines for other soft tissue sarcomas. Radical surgery with complete resection is the primary treatment of choice. Involved margins resection are common because of the invasive and often multifocal nature of angiosarcomas, which confer a worse prognosis. Angiosarcomas have an overall 5 year survival of about 35%. Even with localised disease, the most optimistic survey suggests only 60% of patients survive for more than 5 years, with a median survival of 7 months (Young,2010). However, there are reports of some long-term survivors with metastatic disease, but which prognostic factors are important is unclear.

4.2 Lymphatic metastasis and neck dissection

The incidence of lymph node metastasis of angiosarcoma was found to be 13.5 % (Fong, 2010). Angiosarcoma is particularly prone to nodal metastasis. Prognosis of such metastasis is poor, but certainly not hopeless. Neck dissection is appropriate treatment for isolated metastasis to regional lymph nodes and might provide long-term survival.

5. Synovial sarcoma

Synovial sarcoma is a malignant soft-tissue neoplasm uncommonly found in the head and neck. Although synovial sarcoma is usually found near large joints and bursae of the extremities, it rarely arises from synovial membranes. It accounts for approximately 8% of all soft-tissue sarcomas. Only 10% of all synovial sarcomas occur in the head and neck, and these rarely have an obvious association with synovial structures (Amble et al,1997). Synovial sarcoma were most commonly located in the neck (60%); thus, the most common symptoms were a neck mass and neck pain. Ninety percent of Synovial sarcoma have an identifiable translocation between chromosomes 18 and X that results in the fusion of the SYT gene on chromosome 18 and the SSX-1 or SSX-2 gene on chromosome X (Harb et al, 2007).

5.1 Treatment

As with other soft tissue sarcomas, radical surgery with complete resection is the primary treatment of choice. Unfortunately, up to 50% of Synovial sarcoma recur, usually within 2years. Some 40% metastasis, commonly to lungs and bone and also regional lymph nodes. The best outcome are in childfood patients, in tumors which are <5cm in diameter, have < 10 mitoses/ 10 hpf and no necrosis, and when the tumor is eradicated loccaly. (Christopher et al, 2010)

5.2 Lymph node metastasis and neck dissection

Although not normally a feature of sarcomas, metastasis to regional lymph nodes occurs in 12.5% of cases of synovial sarcoma in the head and neck and 23% of cases in the extremities (Roth et al, 1975). Neck dissection is appropriate treatment for isolated metastasis to regional lymph nodes and may provide long-term survival.

6. Osteosarcoma

Osteosarcoma is the most common primary malignancy of bone. These tumors typically originate in the extremities and the pelvis, with only 6–10% of patients presenting with a head and neck primary tumor (Russell et al, 2003). The mandible and maxilla are the predominate locations of head and neck osteosarcoma (HNOS), although extragnathic bone as well as soft tissues sites may be affected. The peak age of incidence for osteosarcoma outside the head and neck is in the adolescent years. In contrast, HNOS most commonly affects patients in their 30s. Distant metastases have been reported in 10–20% of patients with HNOS, compared with 53–75% of patients with disease arising outside the head and neck. The 5-year, disease-specific survival rate for patients with HNOS has been poor, with most studies reporting survival rates of 23–37%. Management of osteosarcoma outside the head and neck prior to the standardized use of chemotherapy resulted in worse 5-year survival rates of 10–20%.It is widely accepted that wide surgical excision is the mainstay of therapy for patients with HNOS. Adjuvant treatment with radiotherapy and/or chemotherapy also has been administered. For patients with osteosarcoma arising outside the head and neck, surgery also is considered a key component in therapy, but the addition of neoadjuvant and/or adjuvant chemotherapy has improved survival markedly. The Multi-Institution Osteosarcoma Study identified an increase in the 6-year, event-free survival rate from 11% with surgery alone to 61% when chemotherapy was given postoperatively.13 Over the last 2 decades, the standard therapy for patients with non-head and neck osteosarcoma has evolved to routinely include both neoadjuvant and adjuvant chemotherapy. With these regimens, long-term survival rates of 70–80% are being obtained. Whether these same results can be obtained in patients with HNOS is not yet known.

6.1 Treatment

The mainstay of treatment of head and neck osteosarcoma is surgery. Adjuvant postoperative RT is indicated for those with close or positive margins. The role of adjuvant chemotherapy is unclear.

6.2 Lymph node metastasis and neck dissection

The AJCC (2010) definitions of TNM showed that any regional lymph node metastasis (N1) classified to Stage IVB. It suggested to the extremely poor prognosis in front of the neck metastasis of the osteosarcoma. In rare case, Extraskeletal osteosarcoma was present ,That is a high-grade malignant sarcomas defined (1) soft tissue origin and no attachment to the bone or periosteum, (2) a uniform sarcomatous pattern (to exclude the possibility of a mixed malignant mesenchymal tumor), with production of osteoid and/or cartilage matrix. We reported a young patient with highly malignant HNOS, which was excised but was subsequently complicated by local and distant metastases.(Saito et al,2008)

6.3 Case report

A 17-year-old Japanese man with no history of trauma or irradiation was referred to the hospital with complaints of a swelling in the left side of the neck that had been gradually increasing in size. Physical examination showed a smooth, stony hard, mobile mass measuring 24 x 30 mm in the left submandibular region. A computed tomographic scan (figure 3) showed a calcified mass measuring 23 x 18 mm in size, unattached to the hyoid bone or the mandible. The tumor was mildly adherent to the suprahyoid muscles. It was excised along with surrounding muscle. The surgical margin was free of in the direction of the hyoid bone. Three months after the operation, the patient developed massive local recurrence of the tumor. We removed the tumor encased by the surrounding muscles. Postoperatively, the patient received a course of radiotherapy. However, 4 months after the second operation, he developed left facial nerve palsy and complained of sudden hearing loss on the left side. A CT scan showed tumor recurrence in the temporal bone, occupying the middle cranial fossa. The patient and his family selected chemotherapy instead of surgery, but 1month after the start of chemotherapy consisting of Cisplatin 125mg/body and Pirarubicin 60mg/body, the patient developed intracranial hemorrhage and died of hydrocephalus.

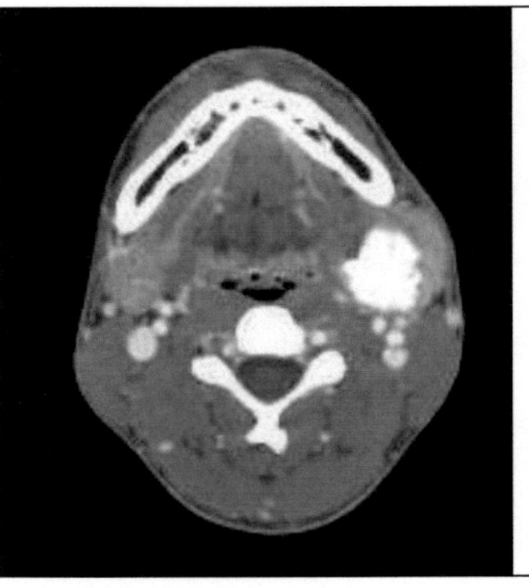

Fig. 3. A case of extraskeletal osteosarcoma of 17-year-old male. (Our experienced case)

7. Chondrosarcoma

Chondrosarcoma is a malignant tumor in which the tumor cells form chondroid (cartilage) but not osteoid. Although chondrosarcoma most commonly arises from either cartilaginous structures or bone derived from chondroid precursors, chondrosarcoma may also arise in areas where cartilage is not normally found. Skull bones were the predominant tissue (59.7%) arose chondrosarcoma. Among these cases were 7.7% originating in the mandible. laryngotracheal cases were about 23.4% in all cases. The other sites were oral cavity, pharynx, and orbit (Koch et al, 2000).

These tumors developing in soft tissue presumably arise from cartilaginous differentiation of primitive mesenchymal cells. Chondrosarcomas develop more commonly in bone than cartilage. However, a sufficiently large number develop from laryngeal cartilage, so that chondrosarcoma is the most common sarcoma developing in the larynx.

It is noteworthy that more than 90% of laryngotracheal chondrosarcoma cases were low grade and occurred in older patients (>50 years). These associations suggest that laryngotracheal tumors represent a form of chondrosarcoma that should be distinguished from cases arising in osseous sites of the head and neck that are more commonly characterized by a younger age and a higher grade. The recognized difficulty in discriminating between the benign laryngeal chondromatous lesions and low-grade chondrosarcomas confounds the interpretation of tumor behavior at this site. It is possible that the large number of low-grade chondrosarcomas identified within the cartilaginous laryngotracheal site may reflect the inclusion of some benign cases erroneously diagnosed as cancer. Despite ongoing study, a widely accepted approach to analysis of cytogenic or proliferative characteristics has yet to surpass grading as an independent predictor of the biologic behavior of chondrosarcoma (Koch et al,2000).

7.1 Treatment

Head and neck chondrosarcomas are generally slow-growing tumors with an indolent course. Yet, owing to the locally aggressive nature and the propensity to recur if not adequately treated, most studies recommend wide en bloc surgical resection as the mainstay of treatment. Conservative resection of low-grade lesions of the larynx has been proven effective in several reports. Organ preservation may be archived with such an approach, which has important functional outcome implications (Hong et al, 2009).

7.2 Lymph node metastasis and neck dissection

In the largest series to date representing 151 cases of chondrosarcoma of the head and neck, Weiss and Bennett noted that "metastasis is not common and generally occurs late in the disease, usually after multiple surgical manipulations."(Weiss & Bennett, 1986) Mark et al stated that "only 1/18 (5%) patients recurred in regional lymph nodes without elective neck treatment, further justifying the accepted approach of not electively treating the neck in head and neck sarcomas."(Mark et al, 1993)

7.3 Case report

A 55-year-old female was referred to us in 2003 because of a 2-years history of hoarseness. She also complained about having dyspnea and had underwent tracheostomy. Direct laryngoscopy revealed a smooth, firm subglottic mass at the subglottis. The CT scan showed a mass that had eroded almost half of the left cricoid cartilage (Figure 4), and the biopsy revealed chondroma. An excision of the tumor and 4/5 cricoid cartilage was resected. A tracheofissure was done at the end of the operation to put a stent T tube in place. Histopathologic examination of the surgical specimen confirmed a grade I chondrosarcoma. 27 months later, direct laryngoscopy was done with no evidence of recurrence. Afterall, we reconstructed the anterior wall of trachea by the costal cartilage. Up until now, the patient has been followed up regularly. In May 2011, 8 years after surgery, she was in perfect health except for a paralysis of the left vocal cord.

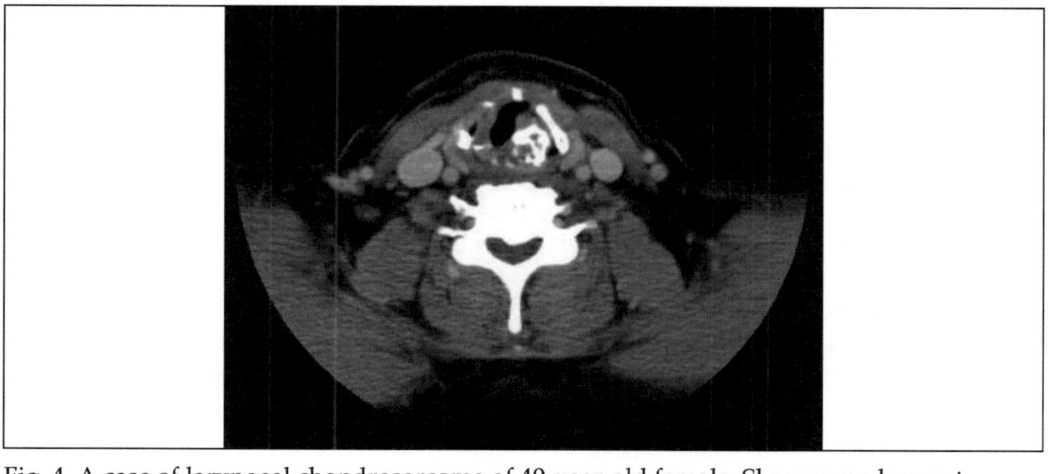

Fig. 4. A case of laryngeal chondrosarcoma of 40-year-old female. She was underwent operation with laryngeal preservation 9 years ago. Now she was free of disease with laryngeal function. (Our experienced case)

8. Ewing's sarcoma

Ewing's sarcoma arising in the head and neck region is extremely rare, comprising 1-4% of all cases of Ewing's sarcoma. Most authors claim a better prognosis for Ewing's sarcoma of the head and neck region as compared to that arising in other anatomic locations. The most commonly affected bones in the head and neck region are the skull, the mandible and the maxilla. There has also been case reports of localized Ewing's sarcoma affecting the orbital roof, the retropharynx and the nasal cavity (Allam et al, 1999).

8.1 Treatment

Surgery after chemotherapy is the current standard of cure. Despite the lack of randomized trials comparing different local treatment modalities in Ewing' Sarcoma, wide surgical resection is considered the treatment of choice. It reduces the local relapse rate, improves the overall survival and may avoid radiotherapy. Ludwig affirms that chemotherapy alone is an ineffective measure in achieving local control of disease (Ludwig, 2008). Thus, it is commonly accepted that an attempt at complete tumour resection should always be made. Nevertheless chemoradiation may be a reasonable alternative to surgery for treatment of tumours that are resectable only with an unacceptable degree of mutilation.

8.2 Lymph node metastasis and neck dissection

Lymphnodes metastasis from Ewing's sarcoma are very rare. The nodal status included as a prognostic indicator in the American Joint Committee on Cancer (AJCC) staging system has even been considered irrelevant by some authors. Considering this, it can be argued that elective neck dissection is not indicated. Nevertheless, as best as we could determine, this argument is not discussed in the literature.

9. Conclusion

Head and neck sarcomas are rare tumors and represent a heterogeneous group of tumours of different histological variants. Subtyping of sarcomas is increasingly important because of the development of biologic response modifiers. Although traditional morphological assessment is the foundation of clinical decision making, immunohistochemistry and molecular biology are useful for diagnosis, prognosis and identification of possible targets for molecular therapy. The management of sarcomas in the head and neck is primarily surgical. Since, in head and neck sarcomas it is difficult to obtain wide margins during surgical treatment, because of anatomic constraints, most patients with locally resectable tumours undergo post-operative irradiation. Modern reconstructive surgery makes more extensively resection possible and may improve local tumour control, while providing acceptable cosmetic and functional results. Adjuvant systemic chemotherapy seems to improve outcome, but its benefit must be weighted against associated toxicities. Survival of patients with head and neck soft tissue sarcoma varies from 50 to 80% and depends on prognostic factors as tumour grade, margin status and tumour size. With further insight into the biology of soft tissue sarcoma and the combination of new treatment options with modern imaging techniques, we will most certainly be able to improve clinical outcome in patients with soft tissue sarcoma in the upcoming years.

10. References

Allam A, El-Husseiny G, Khafaga Y, Kandil A, Gray A, Ezzat A, Schultz H. (1999)Ewing's Sarcoma of the Head and Neck: A Retrospective Analysis of 24 Cases. *Sarcoma.* 3(1):pp.11-5.

Amble FR, Olsen KD, Nascimento AG, Foote RL(1992). Head and neck synovial cell sarcoma. *Otolaryngol Head Neck Surg.* 107(5),Nov,pp.631-7.

Brockstein B (2004). Management of sarcomas of the head and neck. *Curr Oncol Rep.* 6(4),Jul,pp321-327

Callender TA, Weber RS, Janjan N, Benjamin R, Zaher M, Wolf P, el-Naggar A(1995). Rhabdomyosarcoma of the nose and paranasal sinuses in adults and children. *Otolaryngol Head Neck Surg.* 112(2),Feb,pp.252-257.

Costa MJ, Campman SC, Davis RL, Howell LP (1996). Fine-needle aspiration cytology of sarcoma: retrospective review of diagnostic utility and specificity. *Diagn Cytopathol.* 15(1),Jul,pp23-32.

Christopher D.M.Fletcher, K.Krishnan Unni, Fredrik Mertens (2010).*World Heath Organization Classification of Tumours. Pathology & Genetics Tumours of Soft Tissue and Bone.* 6 Skeletal muscle tumours pp.127-134,IARC

Christopher D.M.Fletcher, K.Krishnan Unni, Fredrik Mertens (2010).*World Heath Organization Classification of Tumours. Pathology & Genetics Tumours of Soft Tissue and Bone.* 9 Tumours of uncertain differentiation pp.200-204,IARC

de Bree R, van der Waal I, de Bree E, Leemans CR(2010). Management of adult soft tissue sarcomas of the head and neck. *Oral Oncol.* 46(11),Nov,pp.786-90

Fong Y, Coit DG, Woodruff JM, Brennan MF(1993). Lymph node metastasis from soft tissue sarcoma in adults. Analysis of data from a prospective database of 1772 sarcoma patients. *Ann Surg.* 217(1),Apr,pp.72-77.

Fyrmpas G, Wurm J, Athanassiadou F, Papageorgiou T, Beck JD, Iro H, Constantinidis J.(2009) Management of paediatric sinonasal rhabdomyosarcoma. *J Laryngol Otol.* 123(9),Sep,pp.990-6.

Gradoni P, Giordano D, Oretti G, Fantoni M, Ferri T(2010). The role of surgery in children with head and neck rhabdomyosarcoma and Ewing's sarcoma. *Surg Oncol.* 19(4),Dec,pp.e103-9.

Harb WJ, Luna MA, Patel SR, Ballo MT, Roberts DB, Sturgis EM(2007). Survival in patients with synovial sarcoma of the head and neck: association with tumor location, size, and extension. *Head Neck.* 29(8),Aug,pp.731-40.

Hong P, Taylor SM, Trites JR, Bullock M, Nasser JG, Hart RD (2009). Chondrosarcoma of the head and neck: report of 11 cases and literature review. *J Otolaryngol Head Neck Surg.* 38(2),Apr,pp.279-85

Jones C, Liu K, Hirschowitz S, Klipfel N, Layfield LJ (2002). Concordance of histopathologic and cytologic grading in musculoskeletal sarcomas: can grades obtained from analysis of the fine-needle aspirates serve as the basis for therapeutic decisions? *Cancer.* 96(2),Apr,pp83-91.

Koch BB, Karnell LH, Hoffman HT, Apostolakis LW, Robinson RA, Zhen W, Menck HR(2000). National cancer database report on chondrosarcoma of the head and neck. *Head Neck.* 22(4),Jul,pp.408-25.

Ludwig JA(2008). Ewing sarcoma: historical perspectives, current state-of-the-art, and opportunities for targeted therapy in the future. *Curr Opin Oncol.* 20(4),Jul,pp.412-8.

Mark RJ, Tran LM, Sercarz J, Fu YS, Calcaterra TC, Parker RG(1993). Chondrosarcoma of the head and neck. The UCLA experience, 1955-1988. *Am J Clin Oncol.* 16(3),Jun,pp.232-7.

Montgomery PQ, Peter H.Rhys Evans, Patrick J.Gullane (2009). *Principles and Practice of Head and Neck Surgery and Oncology.Second Edition.* Sarcomas of Head and Neck. ,pp.455-479,Informa healthcare

Moretti G, Guimarães R, Oliveira KM, Sanjar F, Voegels RL(2010). Rhabdomyosarcoma of the head and neck: 24 cases and literature review. *Braz J Otorhinolaryngol.* 76(4),Aug,pp.533-7

Schalow EL, Broecker BH(2003). Role of surgery in children with rhabdomyosarcoma. *Med Pediatr Oncol.* 41(1),Jul,pp.1-6

Rodeberg DA, Paidas CN, Lobe TL, Brown K, Andrassy RJ, Crist WM, Wiener ES. (2002). Surgical Principles for Children/Adolescents With Newly Diagnosed Rhabdomyosarcoma: A Report from the Soft Tissue Sarcoma Committee of the Children's Oncology Group. *Sarcoma,*6(4),pp.111-22.

Roth JA, Enzinger FM, Tannenbaum M(1975). Synovial sarcoma of the neck: a followup study of 24 cases. *Cancer.* 35(4),Apr,pp.1243-53.

Saito Y, Miyajima C, Nakao K, Asakage T, Sugasawa M(2008). Highly malignant submandibular extraskeletal osteosarcoma in a young patient. *Auris Nasus Larynx.* 35(4),Dec,pp.576-8.

Smith RB, Apostolakis LW, Karnell LH, Koch BB, Robinson RA, Zhen W, Menck HR, Hoffman HT(2003). National Cancer Data Base report on osteosarcoma of the head and neck. *Cancer.* 98(8),Oct,pp.1670-80.

Weiss WW Jr, Bennett JA(1986). Chondrosarcoma: a rare tumor of the jaws. *J Oral Maxillofac Surg.* 44(1),Jan,pp.73-9.

Wong SL(2008). Diagnosis and management of desmoid tumors and fibrosarcoma. J Surg Oncol.97(6),May,pp.554-8.

Wurm J, Constantinidis J, Grabenbauer GG, Iro H(2005). Rhabdomyosarcomas of the nose and paranasal sinuses: treatment results in 15 cases. Otolaryngol Head Neck Surg. 133(1), Jul,pp.42-50.

Young RJ, Brown NJ, Reed MW, Hughes D, Woll PJ(2010). Angiosarcoma. *Lancet Oncol.* 11(10), Oct,pp.983-91.

10

Rare Malignant Tumors of the Parotid Glands: Oncocytic Neoplasms

Fatih Oghan[1], Tayfun Apuhan[2] and Ali Guvey[1]
[1]*Dumlupinar University, Faculty of Medicine, Department of Otorhinolaryngology Head and Neck Surgery, Central Campus,Kutahya*
[2]*Abant Izzet Baysal University, Faculty of Medicine, Department of Otorhinolaryngology Head and Neck Surgery, Golkoy, Bolu,*
Turkey

1. Introduction

Salivary gland neoplasms are a rare group of tumors; the annual incidence rate is 1 in 100,000 individual, comprising about 3% of all head and neck neoplasms [4]. The mean age of patients with salivary gland tumors is 45 years, peaking in the sixth and seventh decades of life. Benign salivary gland tumors occur more frequently in females, while malignant tumors are slightly more frequent in males. The parotid gland is the most frequent site - about 70% of cases. About 80% of parotid tumors are benign and 64 to 80% of all primary salivary gland epithelial tumors involve the parotid gland, mostly located in the superficial lobe [5].

Oncocytic neoplasms comprise a group of rare tumours of the parotid glands, and their incidence represents approximately 1% of parotid neoplasms [1]. Histologically they are classified according to the new World Health Organization classification in three distinct types, namely oncocytosis, oncocytoma and oncocytic carcinoma [2]. Oncocytomas usually occur in the elderly and affect the parotid glands in 80% [3]. Pathologically, oncocytoma is described as a well circumscribed mass, composed of layers of oncocytes (small round nucleus, micro-granular, eosinophilic cytoplasm). Oncocytes are large, granular, eosinophilic epithelial cells mainly found in glandular tissue, including that of the salivary glands and thyroid. Oncocytomas that originate from oncocytes are very rare neoplasms that account for less than 1% of all salivary gland tumors [4].

Oncocytic carcinomas are even more uncommon; they represent 11% of all oncocytic salivary gland neoplasms, 0.5% of all epithelial salivary gland malignancies and 0.18% of all epithelial salivary gland tumors [5, 10]. The terms oncocytic carcinoma, oncocytic adenocarcinoma, malignant oncocytoma and malignant oxyphilic adenoma are synonymous [6]. Besides these defined neoplasms, there are other entities that are not well identified oncocytic changes of the parotid gland, such as oncocytic metaplasia, diffuse oncocytosis, nodular oncocytosis and multifocal nodular oncocytic hyperplasia and also oncocytic metaplasia within other salivary gland tumors such as the Warthin's tumor [7].

While the diagnosis of these lesions is usually straightforward, the histologic distinction between nodular oncocytosis and oncocytoma is admittedly rather arbitrary in certain cases.

Many pathologists believe the presence of a single, well-circumscribed and at least partially encapsulated nodule favors the diagnosis of oncocytoma while multiple, unencapsulated nodules distributed in a lobular configuration favors nodular oncocytosis [25]. Even more confusing is the designation of oncocytoma arising in oncocytosis to describe a dominant often encapsulated nodule in the background of oncocytosis. This distinction, however, is academic and of little to no clinical or prognostic significance. More important is the distinction of these lesions from their malignant counterparts, oncocytic carcinomas, as well as the oncocytic variants of other salivary gland carcinomas and metastatic lesions with oncocytic morphology. Also, oncocytic cells have been reported to occur in mucoepidermoid carcinoma (MEC); in addition, a rare variant of MEC known as oncocytic MEC has been described in the last decade [16-19]. These tumors are composed exclusively of oncocytic cells arranged in nests and sheets in sclerotic stroma with variable number of chronic inflammatory cells [19]. The majority of the oncocytic MEC described in the literature as lack of or containing minimal squamous /epidermoid cells. On re-review we believe, based on the criteria described by Weinreb et.al, 5 of 10 cases represent MEC containing oncocytic cells as one the cellular components while 5 of 10 cases represent true oncocytic variant of MEC [19]. We believe that the most helpful features in differentiating MEC containing oncocytic cells from other salivary gland lesions in FNA specimens is the presence of extracellular mucin, mucous cells and pseudo-goblet/clear cells.

Many types of benign and malignant salivary gland tumors can have foci of oncocytic cells. If the oncocytic component comprises a small portion of the lesion the differential diagnosis is not a challenge. Oncocytomas may be unencapsulated and exhibit atypical nuclear changes which may make a distinction from oncocytic carcinoma complicated. In comparison with those two entities oncocytic carcinomas usually have considerably greater mitotic figures, cellular pleomorphism (fig. 1) and most importantly unequivocal evidence infiltration into surrounding tissues (fig. 2). Etit et al [20] showed that a tumor titled as oncocytic Carcinoma ex pleomorphic adenoma composed exclusively of malignant oncocytic cells with extensive infiltration into the surrounding tissues including muscle, vascular and perineural invasion with 23 metastatic cervical lymph nodes. A total parotidectomy with a functional neck dissection was performed. Macroscopically, two distinct tumors were identified; one located in the superficial lobe and the other located in the deep lobe. Microscopically the tumor in the superficial lobe exhibited a tumor composed of large, round, polyhedral cells arranged in small clusters, with isolated individual cells, and occasionally, solid sheets. On hematoxylin and eosin slides, cells had abundant, finely granular, eosinophilic cytoplasm (fig. 3). Many of the oncocytic cells had pleomorphic, medium or large nuclei with an eosinophilic irregular, macronucleoli. Necrosis and extensive lymphovascular tumoral thrombi were noted, but no comedonecrosis, tubular, cribriform or papillary areas were seen. Focally, oncocytic changes were noted in residual normal salivary gland parenchyma. In the deep lobe, in addition to the neoplastic oncocytes, there was close association of various epithelial cell types some forming ductal structures and myxoid mesenchymal-like stroma of a typical pleomorphic adenoma. In their case, 50% of the tumor in the deep lobe was histologically compatible with pleomorphic adenoma with oncocytic carcinoma, while 100% of the tumor in the superficial lobe was oncocytic carcinoma. The clinical significance of oncocytic carcinoma to the prognosis of oncocytic Carcinoma ex pleomorphic adenoma has not known. The tumour may show positive immunoreactivity for AE-1/AE-3, CK-7, CEA, EMA and p63.

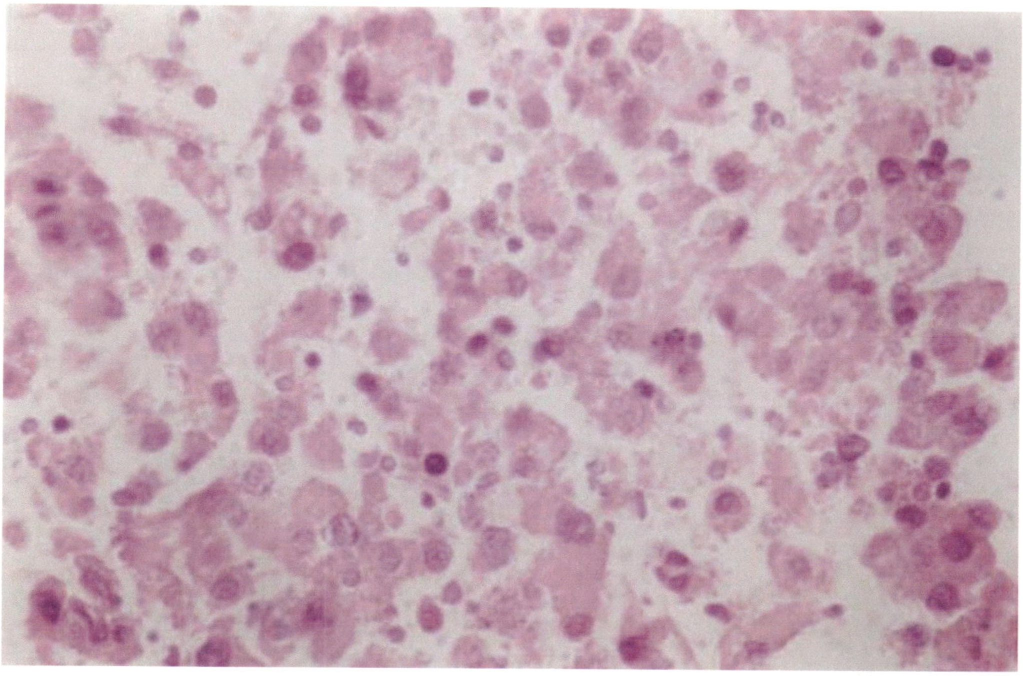

Fig. 1. The tumor consists of oncocytes only (H&E, original magnification, x200)

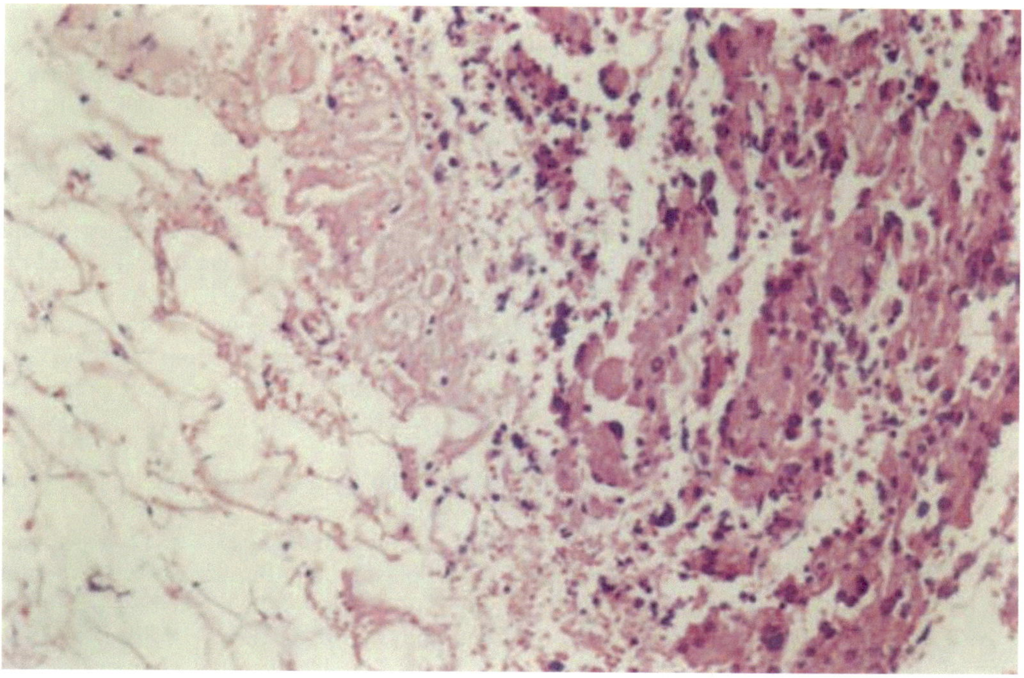

Fig. 2. Tumor cells infiltrating the surrounding adipose tissue are seen (H&E, original magnification, x100)

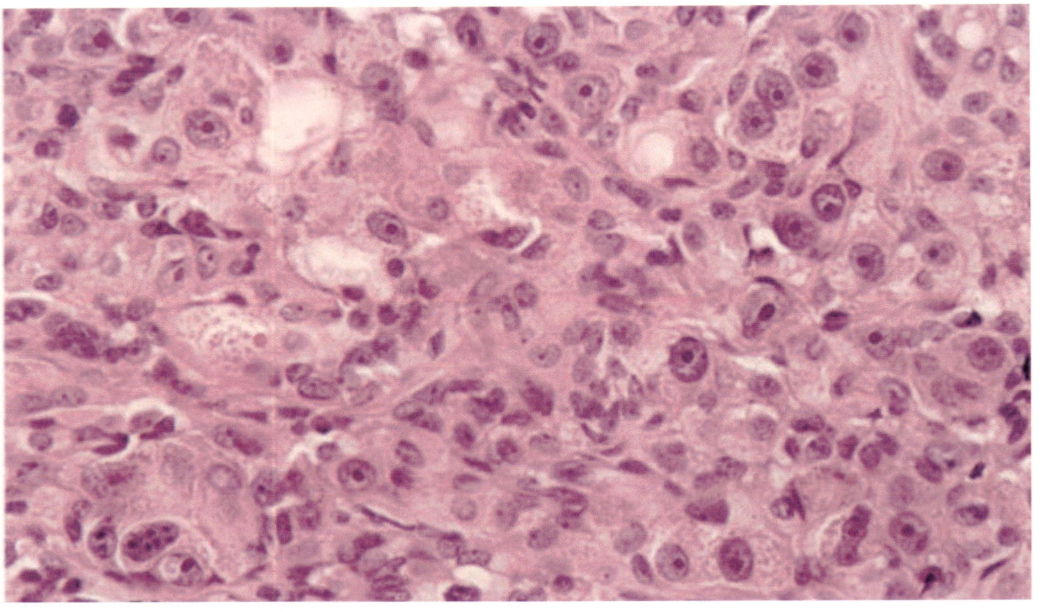

(*Figure 3 is from Prof. Dr Yan Gao, permission was taken)

Fig. 3. The tumor cells having eosinophilic granular cytoplasm and round vesicular nuclei (sometimes double nuclei), often with big and red nucleoli. (H&E)

Epithelial-myoepithelial carcinoma (EMCa) is an uncommon, biphasic salivary gland malignancy composed of ductal epithelial cells and myoepithelial cells with a broad morphologic spectrum. Among these variants was the oncocytic or oncocytic-sebaceous EMCa (OEMCa), which was initially described by Savera and Salama in 2005 [21]. This variant that was defined by prominent oncocytic change in the ductal and/or myoepithelial component and sebaceous elements populated 8% of all EMCa [22]. The cells in this variant are true oncocytes because the prominent granular, eosinophilic cytoplasm is constituted by abundant mitochondria. However, unlike the oncocytes in OEMCa, apocrine epithelial-myoepithelial carcinoma cells could only be considered "oncocytoid" because they did not quite show the same degree of granularity or abundant mitochondria by histochemical or immunohistochemical stains. Their eosinophilia is likely a result of a combination of factors: protein content, secretory vacuoles, with perhaps a minor contribution from mitochondria. These cells showed periapical snouts, vacuolated cytoplasm, and nuclei with prominent central nucleoli and were also positive for androgen receptor (AR), which is typically expressed in salivary duct carcinoma.

Oncocytic carcinoma may occur in many sites in addition to the salivary glands, including the nasal and thoracic cavities, ovary, kidney, thyroid gland, breast and parathyroid.

Oncocytic salivary gland carcinoma is uncommon representing only 0.05–0.4% of salivary gland neoplasms and about 5% of oncocytic neoplasms [3]. Similar to their benign counterparts, nearly 80% occur in the parotid gland. Interestingly, the majority is presumed to arise in a preexisting oncocytoma but they also may occur de novo [14,15]. Diagnostic criteria for salivary gland oncocytic carcinoma include destructive invasion of adjacent salivary or non-salivary tissue, perineural and/or vascular invasion, and metastases. Oncocytic carcinoma is an unusual proliferation of cytomorphologically malignant oncocytes and adenocarcinomatous architecture phenotypes mainly found in glandular tissue [8]. The terms oncocytic carcinoma, oncocytic adenocarcinoma, malignant oncocytoma and malignant oxyphilic adenoma are synonymous. Its malignant nature is distinguished from oncocytoma by abnormal morphological features and infiltrative growth [3]. The majority of oncocytic carcinoma cases have occurred in the parotid glands, but tumors that involved the submandibular gland and minor glands of the palate have also been described [11]. Also, oncocytic carcinoma of the submandibular gland has only been reported in 11 cases [23]. Fine needle aspiration is the procedure of choice for making a diagnosis in the majority of cases, although its sensitivity is reported to be only 29%, in the oncocytic carcinoma. Rarity of the disease, sampling error and lack of interpreter experience are account for the majority of pitfalls. The oncocytic nature of the tumor cells is confirmed with special methods, such as histochemical or immunohistochemical stains [8]. Necrosis, peri-neural spread, pleomorphism, intravascular invasion, and distant metastasis to the cervical lymph nodes, kidneys, lungs, and mediastinum are the main features of this high-grade malignant tumor [8].

Surgical management with radical or superficial parotidectomy represents the cornerstone of therapy [3]. Probably, there is no need for chemotherapy and/or irradiation, given the benign nature and slow growth rate of the tumour; recurrence is less than 20%, mainly because of incomplete surgical resection. Criteria for the diagnosis of malignancy in salivary oncocytic tumors include: (1) local lymph node metastasis; (2) distant metastasis; (3) peri-neural, vascular or lymphatic invasion; (4) frequent mitoses and cellular pleomorphism with extensive invasion and destruction of adjacent structures [12]. Distant metastasis is very rare. For instance, only one case of oncocytic carcinoma arising in the submandibular gland with disseminated bone metastases was reported in the literature [24]. Local recurrence was also considered as one of the characteristics of oncocytic carcinoma. According to the WHO Histological Typing of Salivary Gland Tumors (2005) [29], two criteria are necessary to establish the diagnosis of oncocytic carcinoma. Firstly, the tumor cells must be identified as oncocytes. Secondly, the diagnosis of malignancy should be based not only on cellular and nuclear pleomorphism, but also on local infiltration and metastasis. Oncocytic carcinoma can be differentiated from benign oncocytoma by the presence of a connective tissue capsule in the latter. Moreover, compared to oncocytoma, oncocytic carcinoma usually shows a greater mitotic activity and more nuclear pleomorphism.

This tumor is predominantly composed of round or polyhedral cells arranged in small clusters and occasional solid sheets. Cells have abundant eosinophilic cytoplasm, a result of excessive numbers of mitochondria [8]. Histochemical and immunohistochemical procedures are also essential for the differential diagnosis [11]. Although not commonly used, it has been reported that anti-mitochondrial antibody is highly specific and sensitive to confirm the oncocytic nature of the granular cytoplasm [13]. FNAC is less sensitive for oncocytic neoplasms, perhaps due to the rarity of these tumors and diagnostic pitfalls previously associated with FNAC (for example, sampling errors and overinterpretation of paucicellular specimens) [3]. Approximately one-third of patients with oncocytic carcinoma of the parotid develop a painful mass or experience facial paralysis. The skin overlying the gland is occasionally discolored or wrinkled [8]. Diagnosis is usually made 1 to 2 years after the onset of disease [4]. For clinicians, the differentiation of oncocytic carcinomas from benign oncocytic neoplasms is quite important. Histologically, oncocytic carcinomas have an infiltrative and at times vascular- or neuroinvasive growth pattern. Histochemically,

PTAH staining distinctly illustrate positive, small, dark-blue cytoplasmic granules, which represent mitochondria. Brandwein and Huvos especially recommended the use of prolonged (48 h) PTAH staining [30]. It has also been reported that immunohistochemistry using an anti-mitochondrial antibody is a highly sensitive and specific method for identifying the mitochondria by light microscopy [13]. This procedure is easy to perform and readily available for the specimens embedded in paraffin which would otherwise not be appropriate for analysis by electron microscopy.

Immuno-phenotypically, tumour shows intense immunoreactivity for mitochondria, CK5/6, CK8/18 (fig. 4), CK10/13, CK19, and EMA, whereas there is no reactivity documented for SMA or S-100 (fig. 5-7) [28]. In addition, there is an increased expression of MIB-1 antibody against Ki-67 antigen in contrast to benign oncocytomas (fig. 8). This finding helps in the differentiation of oncocytic carcinomas from both benign oncocytomas and highly malignant oncocytic carcinomas [7]. Oncocytic lesions are characterized by cells with an atypical accumulation of mitochondria (fig. 9). This accumulation has been recognized as a compensatory mechanism to intrinsic functional defects of these organelles, resulting in energy production impairment and increased generation of reactive oxygen species (ROS), including hydrogen peroxide (H2O2). Peroxiredoxin I (Prx I) is a H2O2 scavenging protein and the expression of its yeast homolog was reported to be influenced by mitochondrial function. Demasi et a showed that Prx I is over-expressed in oncocytes regardless of the salivary gland lesion where they appear. Their results suggested that Prx I expression in oncocytes is related to its ability to decompose mitochondrial-derived H2O2 and that it could provide to the cells a protective role in an environment that, by continuously producing potential DNA-damaging ROS, predisposes to genome instability and cellular transformation [31].

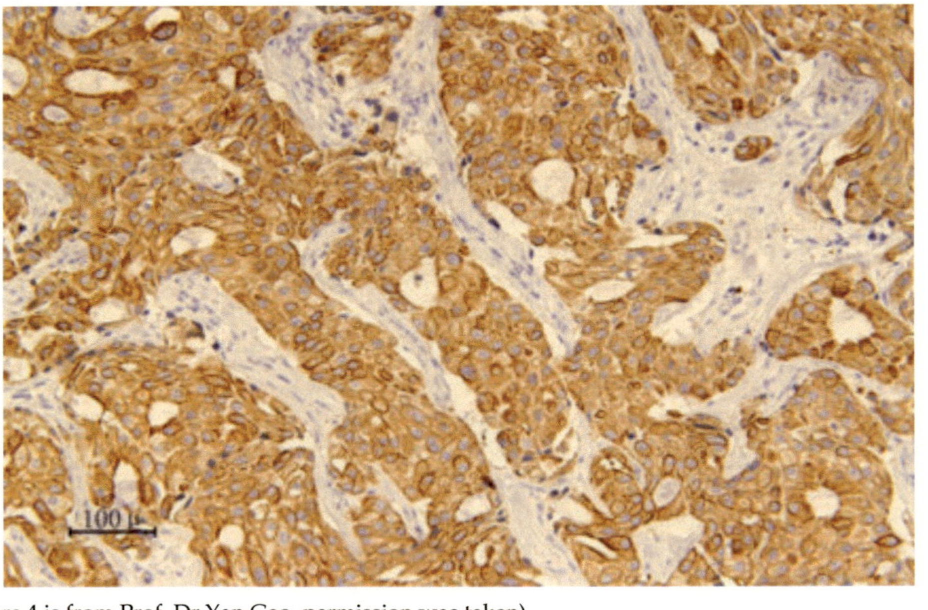

(*Figure 4 is from Prof. Dr Yan Gao, permission was taken)

Fig. 4. Immunohistochemical reactivity of the tumor cells for CK8/18.

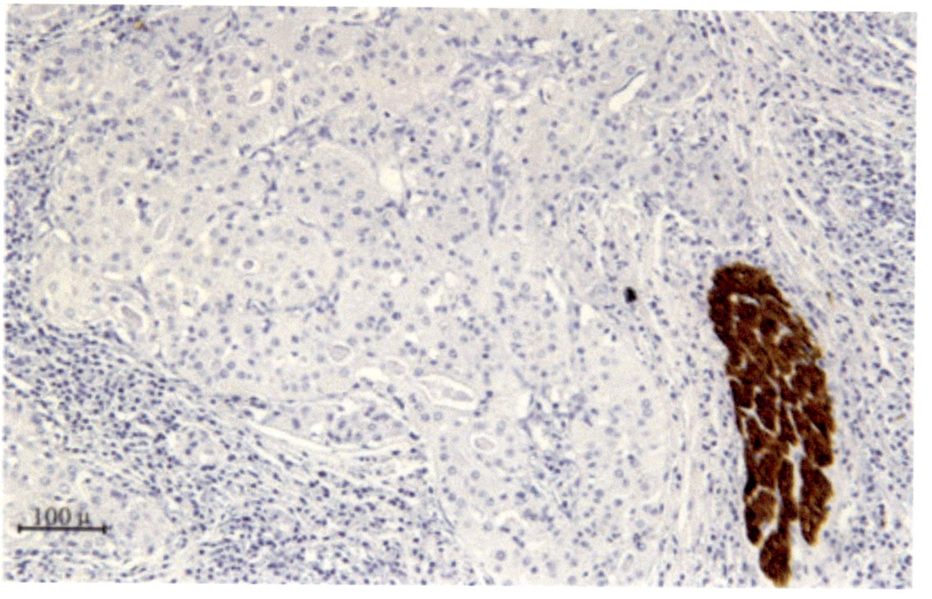

(*Figure 5 is from Prof. Dr Yan Gao, permission was taken)

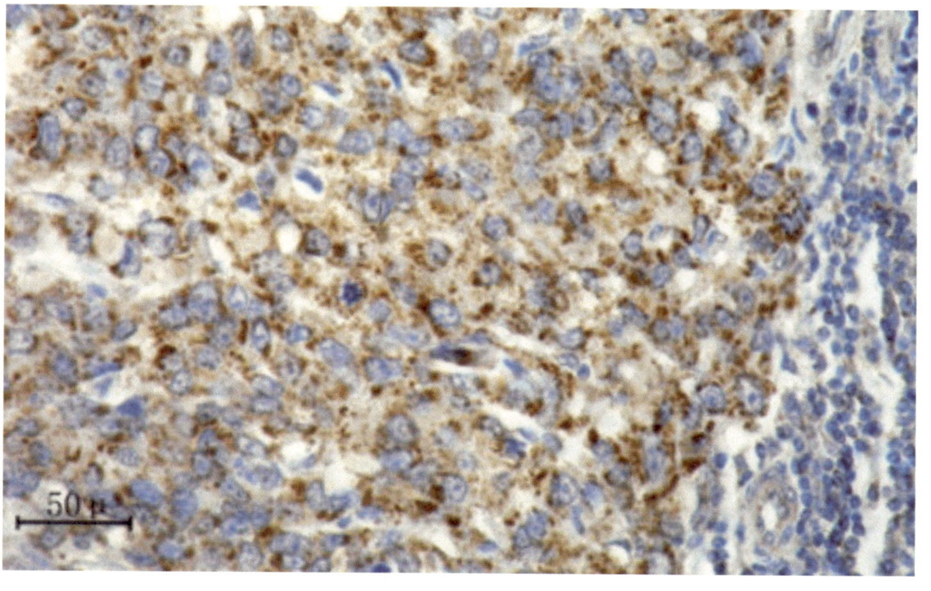

(*Figure 6 is from Prof. Dr Yan Gao, permission was taken)

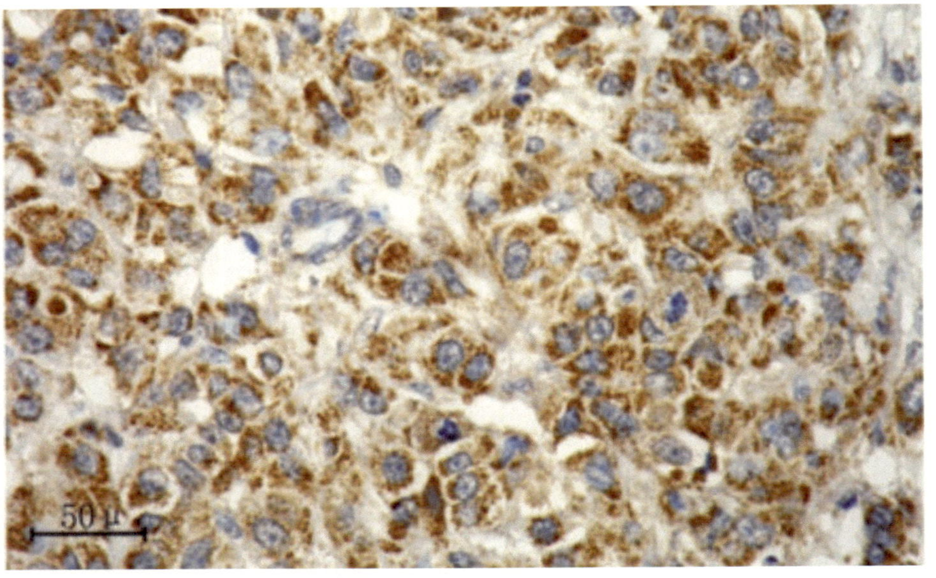

(*Figure 7 is from Prof. Dr Yan Gao, permission was taken)

Fig. 5-7. No S-100 reactivity in tumor cells. Oncocytes in both lymph nodes with metastasis (5) and primary foci (6) have intense granular cytoplasmic immunoreactivity for anti-mitochondria immunostaining (7).

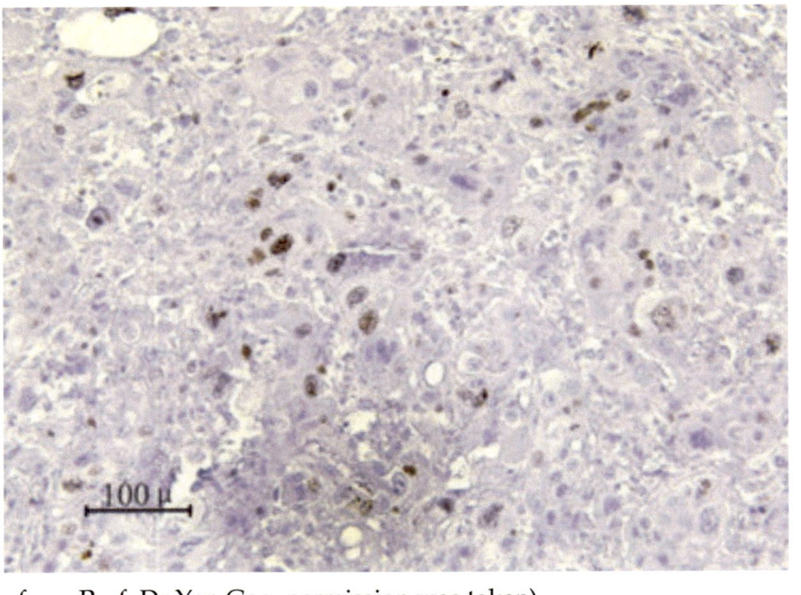

(*Figure 8 is from Prof. Dr Yan Gao, permission was taken)

Fig. 8. Ki-67 positive nuclear staining in malignant oncocytes.

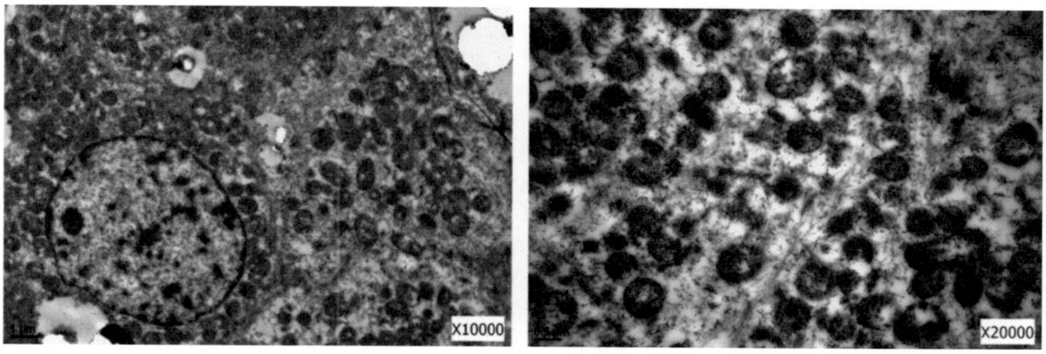

(*Figure 9 is from Prof. Dr Yan Gao, permission was taken)

Fig. 9. Electron microscopy demonstrating numerous mitochondria in the cytoplasm of the tumor cells. (left, x10,000; right, x20,000).

Occasionally, separation of primary salivary oncocytic lesions can be problematic as other salivary gland tumors can demonstrate both oncocytic and clear cell change. Clear cell and/or oncocytic change is either characteristic or present as a common variant in clear cell carcinoma, sebaceous adenoma/carcinoma, pleomorphic adenoma, myoepithelioma, myoepithelial carcinoma, acinic cell carcinoma, epithelial-myoepithelial carcinoma and mucoepidermoid carcinoma. To add to the diagnostic dilemma, metastases to the head and neck region can manifest as oncocytic and/or clear cell lesions. The prototypical metastasis that can masquerade as oncocytoma/oncocytosis is metastatic renal cell carcinoma (RCC). Both lesions can be composed of oncocytic and/or clear cells and both can have similar architectural grown patterns, lumen formation, and vascularized stroma. Although immunohistochemistry panels have been used to aid with this differential, significant overlap in staining limits their usefulness [26]. McHugh et al anecdotally noted that p63 immunohistochemical expression occurs in oncocytomas but not in metastatic RCC to the head and neck [27]. Besides oncocytomas, other tumors are also considered to distinguish from OC. Acinic cell adenocarcinoma can be differentiated from OC since the cytoplasmic granules in acinic cell adenocarcinoma are amphophilic or basophilic and the patterns of growth can be microcystic or papillary. Salivary duct carcinoma, in contrast to OC, usually forms duct-like spaces with papillary and cribriform growth and often shows comedo- like necrosis. In the meantime, the presence of numerous mitochondria in the cytoplasm of the oncocytes that is confirmed on ultrastructural examination is not found in the neoplastic cells from other malignancies mentioned above, which can be considered for adjuvant diagnosis. However, the processes of fixation or embedding of specimens for light microscopy often destroy the fine structure of organelle in the cytoplasm so that it is difficult to observe mitochondria clearly.

Management and treatment of oncocytic carcinomas is not well established due to the low incidence of this tumor type. It consists of surgical intervention and radiotherapy, although the efficacy of radiotherapy is unclear. Surgery especially radical resection is the widely accepted treatment for OC. When the tumor invades the facial nerve, the nerve should be sacrificed in principle. Immediate nerve grafting for reconstruction of facial nerve defect could be performed. Goode and Corio [14] reported 4 cases treated only by conservative surgery all recurred after the operation, three of which metastasized. Furthermore, many cases described in the literature were treated with surgery including neck dissection.

Radiation does not appear to alter favorably the biological behavior of this tumor. Prophylactic neck dissection may be indicated for tumors that are larger than 2 cm in diameter [14]. The prognosis of oncocytic carcinomas is not well known because of their low incidence. Further investigation of the prognosis of patients with oncocytic carcinoma of the parotid gland is warranted as more cases are reported. Nakada et al. reported 23 cases of OC with cervical lymph node metastasis in a review of 42 cases [15]. The patients ranged in age from 30 to 91 years (mean: 58). The analysis of 31 reported cases with information regarding local lymph node and distant metastases and clinical course revealed that nine of ten patients who died of disease had distant metastases, while seven of these ten patients had local lymph node involvement. In contrast, none of 21 living patients had distant metastases, and 11 of these had only local lymph node involvement. Therefore, they concluded that distant metastasis appeared to be the most important prognostic feature of oncocytic carcinoma; local lymph node metastasis was not necessarily a critical factor in the overall prognosis.

Goode and Corio [14] reported that tumors smaller than 2 cm in diameter appeared to be associated with a better prognosis than those that were larger. It has been suggested that elected neck dissection be indicated when the tumor size is larger than 2 cm or the histopathologic features suggest the tumor spreads to the cervical lymph nodes. Adjuvant radiotherapy has also been used for the treatment of oncocytic carcinoma [6, 14, 15, 23]. In Zhou et al [28] study, 5 of 12 patients received radiotherapy, of whom two had multiple metastases and died of disease about 1 year after initial treatment, 2 patients are alive with disease 6 and 42 months after treatment but both with recurrence occurred, and only one is alive without evidence of disease 77 months after treatment. Altogether, for the extensive tumors, radical resection combined with elective neck dissection may be the first choice for treatment, while the role of radiotherapy or chemotherapy is still controversial. It seems clear from these studies that patients who undergo more aggressive initial surgery have a significantly better overall prognosis. I preferred a close follow-up to an elective neck dissection, and reserved the neck dissection for a recurrence.

In summary, oncocytic carcinomas of salivary gland origin are high-grade tumors with local recurrences, regional or distant metastases, diagnosis of which based on a combination of clinical and histopathological features. Immunohistochemistry for mitochondria is considered helpful for the adjuvant diagnosis. Complete surgical excision is the treatment of choice while the role of radiotherapy or chemotherapy is still controversial, and careful long-term follow-up is necessary.

2. References

[1] Stomeo F, Meloni F, Bozzo C, Fois V, Pastore A. Bilateral oncocytoma of the parotid gland. Acta Otolaryngol 2006;126:324-326.

[2] Seifert G. Tumour-like lesions of the salivary glands. The new WHO classification. Pathol Res Pract 1992;188:836-846.

[3] Capone RB, Ha PK, Westra WH, Pilkington TM, Sciubba JJ, Koch WM, Cummings CW. Oncocytic neoplasms of the parotid gland: a 16-year institutional review. Otolaryngol Head Neck Surg 2002;126:657-662.

[4] Ellis GL, Auclair PL. Tumors of the salivary glands. In: Atlas of tumor pathology, 3rd series, fascicle 17. Armed Forces Institute of Pathology, Washington, DC, 1996, pp 318–324

[5] Ellis GL, Auclair PL, Gnepp DR, Goode RK. Other malignant epithelial neoplasms. In: Surgical pathology of the salivary glands. In: Ellis GL, Auclair PL, Gnepp DR (eds) Philadelphia, W. Saunders, 1991, pp 455–488

[6] Cinar U, Vural C, Basak T, Turgut S. Oncocytic carcinoma of the parotid gland: report of a new case. Ear Nose Throat J 2003;82:699–701

[7] Alberty J, August C, Stoll W. Oncocytic neoplasms of the parotid gland. Differential diagnosis, clinical course and review of the literature. HNO 2001;49:109–117

[8] Ellis GL, Auclair PL: Malign epithelial neoplasms. In: Tumors of the salivary glands. Atlas of Tumor Pathology. 4 edition. Washington, DC: Armed Forces Institute of Pathology; 2008, 173-439

[9] Barnes L, Eveson JW, Reichart P, Sidransky D. Pathology and genetics of head and neck tumors. World Health Organization Classification of Tumors Lyon, France: WHO; 2005, 235.

[10] Giordano G, Gabrielli M, Gnetti L, Ferri T. Oncocytic carcinoma of parotid gland: a case report with clinical, immunohistochemical and ultrastructural features. World J Surg Oncol 2006;4:54

[11] Guclu E, Oghan F, Ozturk O, Alper M, Egeli E. A rare malignancy of the parotid gland: oncocytic carcinoma. Eur Arch Otorhinolaryngol 2005;262:567-569.

[12] Gray SR, Cornog JL Jr, Seo IS. Oncocytic neoplasms of salivary glands: a report of fifteen cases including two malignant oncocytomas. Cancer 1976;38:1306-1317.

[13] Shintaku M, Honda T. Identification of oncocytic lesions of salivary glands by anti-mitochondrial immunohistochemistry. Histopathology 1997;31:408-411.

[14] Goode RK, Corio RL. Oncocytic adenocarcinoma of salivary glands. Oral Surg Oral Med Oral Pathol 1988;65:61–66

[15] Nakada M, Nishizaki K, Akagi H, Masuda Y, Yoshino T. Oncocytic carcinoma of the submandibular gland: a case report and literature review. J Oral Pathol Med 1998;27:225–228

[16] Brannon RB and Willard CC. Oncocytic mucoepidermoid carcinoma of parotid gland origin. Oral Surg Oral Med Oral Pathol Oral Radiol Endod. 2003;96(6): 727–733

[17] Corcione L, Giordano G, Gnetti L, Multinu A, Ferrari S. Oncocytic mucoepidermoid carcinoma of a submandibular gland: a case report and review of the literature. Int J Oral Maxillofac Surg 2007;36(6):560–563

[18] Salih Deveci M, Deveci G, Gunhan O, Finci R. Oncocytic mucoepidermoid carcinoma of the parotid gland: report of a case with DNA ploidy analysis and review of the literature. Pathol Int, 2000;50: 905–909

[19] Weinreb I, Seethala RR, Perez-Ordonez B, Chetty R, Hoschar AP, Hunt JL. Oncocytic mucoepidermoid carcinoma: clinicopathologic description in a series of 12 cases. Am J Surg Pathol 2009;33: 409–416

[20] Etit D, Tan A, Bayol U, Altinel D, Cumurcu S, Cukurova I. Oncocytic carcinoma ex pleomorphic adenoma. Head Neck Pathol. 2010;4(1):49-52.

[21] Savera AT, Salama ME. Oncocytic epithelial-myoepithelial carcinoma of the salivary gland: an underrecognized morphologic variant. Mod Pathol. 2005; 18(suppl 1):217A.

[22] Seethala RR, Barnes EL, Hunt JL. Epithelial-myoepithelial carcinoma: a review of the clinicopathologic spectrum and immunophenotypic characteristics in 61 tumors of

the salivary glands and upper aerodigestive tract. Am J Surg Pathol. 2007;31(1):44–57.

[23] Mizutari K, Naganishi H, Tanaka Y. Oncocytic carcinoma in the submandibular gland: report of a case based on anti-mitochondrial immunohistochemical observations. Auris Nasus Larynx 2005;32:305–308.

[24] Lee JS, Choi JH, Oh YH. Oncocytic carcinoma arising in the submandibular gland with disseminated bone metastases. South Med J. 2009;102(6):659-62.

[25] Palmer TJ, Gleeson MJ, Eveson JW, et al. Oncocytic adenomas and oncocytic hyperplasia of salivary glands: a clinicopathological study of 26 cases. Histopathology 1990;16:487–93

[26] Ozolek JA, Bastacky SI, Myers EN, et al. Immunophenotypic comparison of salivary gland oncocytoma and metastatic renal cell carcinoma. Laryngoscope 2005;115:1097–100

[27] McHugh JB, Hoschar AP, Dvorakova M, et al. p63 Immunohistochemistry Differentiates Salivary Gland Oncocytoma and Oncocytic Carcinoma from Metastatic Renal Cell Carcinoma. Head and Neck Pathol 2007; 1:123–131

[28] Zhou CX, Shi DY, Ma DQ et al. Primary oncocytic carcinoma of the salivary glands: a clinicopathologic and immunohistochemical study of 12 cases. Oral Oncol. 2010;46:773-8.

[29] Sciubba JJ, Shimono M. Oncocytic carcinoma. In: Barnes L, Eveson JW, Reichart D, Sidransky D, editors. World Health Organization classification of tumours pathology and genetics head and neck tumours. Lyon: IARC Press; 2005. p. 235.

[30] Brandwein MS, Huvos AG. Oncocytic tumors of major salivary glands: a study of 68 cases with follow-up of 44 patients. Am J Surg Pathol 1991;15(6): 514–28.

[31] Demasi APD, Furuse C, Altemani A, et al. Peroxiredoxin I is overexpressed in oncocytic lesions of salivary glands. J Oral Pathol Med 2009;38: 514–517

11

Current Concept of Selective Nek Dissection

H. Hakan Coskun
Uludag University School of Medicine, Department of Otolaryngology
Turkey

1. Introduction

It has long been known that the most important prognostic factor of squamous cell carcinoma of the head and neck is the presence of cervical lymph node metastasis. When neck metastases are not managed properly, this will result a decrease the patient's chance of survival. Radical neck dissection has been introduced in the beginning of 1900's as the surgical procedure to remove cervical lymph nodes systematically in an effort to address metastases and been used widely since then. But radical neck dissection was associated with significant morbidity and especially patients with clinically negative neck were suffering from this unnecessary morbidity. Almost 60 years after introduction of radical neck dissection, Suarez (Ferlito & Rinaldo, 2004) presented modified radical neck dissection (often termed as functional neck dissection). Though, the morbidity associated with neck dissection had been reduced by modified radical neck dissection, efforts to further reduce the morbidity continued and in 1985, Byers (Byers, 1985) reported removal of the cervical lymph node levels which are at the greatest risk for metastasis in patients with clinically negative neck, a surgical procedure which will later be called "selective neck dissection" (Robbins et al, 1991). The rationale behind selective neck dissection is removal of certain lymph node groups, which are at risk for occult metastasis, while preserving the functional structures of the neck and the lymph node groups that are not likely to contain metastasis, in an effort to reduce the risk of complications and morbidity associated with neck dissection.

The current and widely used classification of neck dissections has been introduced by a group of authors from the American Head and Neck Society and American Academy of Otolaryngology-Head and Neck Surgery in 2002 (Robbins, 2002). According to this classification, SND refers to selective neck dissection and the removed lymph node groups are depicted in brackets. For example selective neck dissection involving levels II to IV is recorded as SND (II-IV). The committee also recommended the extent of dissection for each anatomic sub-site. For oral cavity cancer, the recommended procedure was SND (I-III), which was formerly called as supraomohyoid neck dissection. It was noted that level IV might be involved in patients with oral tongue cancer and SND (I-IV), which was formerly called as extended supraomohyoid neck dissection, may be warranted in these patients. The recommended procedure for oropharyngeal, hypopharyngeal and laryngeal cancers was SND (II-IV), which was formerly called lateral neck dissection. The committee noted that level IIB involvement was rare in laryngeal and hypopharyngeal cancers, thus SND (IIA,III,IV) would be sufficient, however removal of level IIB was recommended for oropharyngeal cancers. It was also noted that retropharyngeal lymph nodes needed to be addressed for hypopharyngeal cancers. The committee's recommendation for cancer of the midline structures of the anterior lower neck, such as thyroid cancer, advanced glottic and subglottic larynx cancer, advanced piriform sinus cancer, and cervical esophageal/tracheal cancer, was SND (VI), which was formerly called central neck dissection, with or without dissection of other levels. The recommendation for cutaneous malignancies was tailoring the extent of dissection according to the location of the primary tumor.

Recently, the members of International Head and Neck Scientific Group proposed a new classification for neck dissection (Ferlito, 2011). According to this new classification, ND refers to neck dissection and the removed structures and neck levels are depicted in brackets. For example ND (I-V, SCM, IJV, CN XI) is radical neck dissection, ND (II-IV) is lateral neck dissection. The best advantage of this classification is that any modification of neck dissection can be depicted. For example removal of a non-lymphatic structure during a selective neck dissection can be depicted with this classification, which was not possible with previous classifications.

In the last twenty years, it has been recognized that even after selective neck dissections, patients suffer from some degree of morbidity, such as shoulder dysfunction and chylous fistula. Recently, neck dissections more limited than classical selective neck dissections have been introduced and been advocated by many authors to further reduce the morbidity of neck dissections.

2. Extent of surgical removal for selective neck dissection

The extent of neck dissection is a major debate for the last years because limiting the dissection may help to reduce morbidity, avoid complications and reduce operative time, but this has to be done without reducing the efficacy of neck dissection. For clinically N0 or N1 head and neck cancers of various primary sites, radical neck dissection is considered as an overtreatment, because the three functionally important non-lymphatic tissues that are removed during radical neck dissection, the internal jugular vein, spinal accessory nerve and sternocleidomastoid muscle, are rarely involved in the early stages of the neck disease. Furthermore, in N0 and some N1 head and neck cancers, a modified radical neck dissection is also considered unnecessary, because each head and neck site has a well-known lymphatic drainage pathway and metastases outside these pathways are very rare. Thus, only the lymph node levels that are at the highest risk for metastasis are removed and the other levels are left undissected in order to decrease operative morbidity. Today, efforts to improve the functional results of neck dissection are continuing and a new concept of more limited neck dissection is emerging.

2.1 Selective neck dissection for squamous cell carcinoma of the head and neck

2.1.1 Selective neck dissection for oral cavity cancer

The management of oral cavity cancer with clinically N0 neck varies considerably. It has been clearly demonstrated that occult metastases may occur in up to 20 - 44% (Po Wing Yuen, 2002; Fakih, 1989; Jones, 1992; Kligerman, 1994; Sheahan, 2003; Spiro, 1986; Woolgar, 1999; Ross, 2004; Sparano, 2004) of these patients. This finding supports the need for an elective neck dissection but there are still surgeons who prefer the observation policy reserving neck dissection for regional recurrence. In a recent article, Fasunla et al (Fasunla, 2011) reported the results of a meta-analysis comparing elective neck dissection versus observation in clinically N0 oral cavity cancer. They have found that elective neck dissection reduced the rate of disease-specific death. Obviously, elective neck dissection offers a better outcome in terms of survival, but results in unnecessary morbidity in patients who do not have occult metastases. Thus we need to identify the patients who are more likely to have occult metastases and need elective neck dissection. Studies aiming to identify the rate of occult metastases in relation to various risk factors have shown that tumor thickness (depth of tumor invasion) is a very important factor. Though the tumor thickness measurement methods or tumor-thickness cut-off levels vary considerably among studies, uniformly all studies reported that tumors with a thickness of more than a certain level (ranges from 2 to 10 mm, in most studies 4 or 5 mm) are more likely to develop occult metastases (Pentenero, 2005). According to the author of this chapter's experience, almost all patients present with tumors thicker than 4 or 5 mm, thus almost all patients require elective neck dissection.

Though there is general agreement on elective management of the neck, debate continues on the extent of surgery. Many studies have shown that comprehensive (i.e. level I-V) neck dissections result in unnecessary overtreatment. In a prospective multi-institutional study from Brazil (Brazilian Head and Neck Cancer Study Group, 1998), it has been shown that both modified radical and supraomohyoid neck dissections can offer comparable survival and recurrence rates in treatment of clinically N0 oral cavity cancer.

An ideal neck dissection for clinically N0 neck should remove all the lymph node groups, which potentially harbor occult metastases while preserving the non-lymphatic structures along with the lymph node groups that are unlikely to contain occult metastases. It has been demonstrated that level V is rarely involved in oral cavity cancers (Dias, 2006). Furthermore, these rare metastases to level V occur only when other levels are involved and isolated metastasis to level V never happens (Dias, 2006). It has been well-known that levels I,II and III are the most frequently involved levels in oral cavity cancers and removal of these lymph node groups through a level I-III neck dissection (supraomohyoid neck dissection) has been the standard treatment of clinically N0 oral cavity cancer. However, extension of level I-III neck dissection to include level IV (extended supraomohyoid neck dissection) or removal of level IIB is still debatable.

The significance of level IV metastases without involvement of other levels (i.e. skip metastases) is yet to be known. Some authors have demonstrated that rate level IV metastases are high enough to warrant dissection of this level, with a metastasis rate of 15% (De Zinis, 2006, Byers, 1997). Also, Woolgar (Woolgar, 2006) demonstrated that an important proportion of neck recurrences occurred because of skip metastases to levels III or IV, which is a finding that supports extended supraomohyoid neck dissection for prevention of neck recurrences. On the other hand, there are various reports that demonstrate a low incidence of metastases in level IV (Mishra, 2010, Bajwa 2011). These authors have concluded that extension of dissection to include level IV did not offer an advantage for prevention of neck recurrences and level I-III dissection should be the preferred surgical procedure for management of clinically N0 oral cavity cancer (Bajwa, 2011). In the light of the current literature, the management of level IV is not clear in clinically N0 oral cavity cancer; further prospective and multi-center studies are needed.

Studies have shown that metastases to level IIB from oral cavity cancers are rare, occuring at a mean rate of 6% (Paleri, 2008, Lea, 2010). It has been demonstrated that isolated level IIB metastases from oral cavity cancers are exteremely rare (Lea, 2010). But, when other levels, especially level IIA, contain occult metastases, level IIB metastases may occur in up to 22% of the patients (Elsheikh, 2005, Lea, 2010). Interestingly, level IIB metastases are almost always seen in patients with tongue cancer, however other oral cavity primary sites only rarely give rise to level IIB metastases (Elsheikh, 2005, Lea, 2010). When the lesion is located in the retromolar trigone with extension to the anterior pillar, level IIB should be dissected (Ayad, 2009). Although the current literature demonstrates that level IIB metastases from oral cavity cancers are rare, there is not enough evidence to support preservation of level IIB. Prospective, multi-center studies utilizing standardized surgical dissection and specimen processing techniques are required.

Razfar et al (Razfar, 2009), have shown that submandibular gland is rarely involved in early stage (stage I-II) oral cavity cancers and the gland can be preserved during selective neck dissections. It is true that the submandibular gland is not a lymphatic tissue and unless it is directly invaded by the disease, it does not contain malignant disease. However, there are many lymph nodes in the close vicinity of the gland, which are the first echelon lymph nodes of oral cavity. Thus, one should be very carefully remove all the level I lymph nodes while preserving the gland. The gland should not be preserved if the arterial or venous circulation of the gland is damaged or when post-operative radiotherapy is likely.

2.1.2 Selective neck dissection for Laryngeal cancer

In the intrauterine life, glottis and subglottic larynx is derived from tracheobronchial bud, which develops from the sixth branchial arch and is formed by the union of lateral furrows on each side of the tracheobronchial bud. Supraglottic larynx is derived from buccopharyngeal bud, which develops from third and fourth branchial arches without a midline union. Blood and lymph vessels develop along with these compartments. So, supraglottic and glottic-sublottic compartments have different lymphatic drainage pathways. Supraglottic larynx drains bilaterally into the upper and middle jugular lymph nodes, whereas glottic and subglottic regions drain into lower jugular, prelaryngeal and pretracheal lymph nodes. Supraglottic larynx has a rich lymphatic network and metastasis can occur even in the early stages of cancer, however vocal folds have sparse lymphatic channels, so metastases from early glottic lesions are rare (Armstrong, 1995). This basic knowledge provides a basis for planning of neck dissection in relation to the primary tumor.

Lateral neck dissection (SND II–IV) has been used widely in the past twenty years for management of the neck in clinically N0 laryngeal cancer because it has been demonstrated that metastases of laryngeal cancer usually occurs in these levels and levels I and V are rarely involved (Robbins, 2002, Kowalski, 1995, Jones, 1994, Ferlito, 2001). SND II–IV is very effective in treating occult metastases and in a previous study from the author of this chapter's department, it has been demonstrated that a neck recurrence rate as low as 1.7% can be achieved after SND II–IV (Erisen, 2001).

Although SND provides excellent oncological results, functional outcome after SND II-IV is not as good as expected. A prospective study from the author of this chapter's department has demonstrated that there is dysfunction of the spinal accessory nerve after SND (Erisen, 2004). Koybasioglu et al (Koybasioglu, 2000) have also shown that spinal accessory nerve function is impaired after SND. The most possible reason of dysfunction is retraction of the spinal accessory nerve during clearance of sublevel IIB. Numerous studies have shown that the incidence of metastasis in sublevel IIB is very low. In the prospective studies, including one study by the author of this chapter, analyzing the rate of sublevel IIB metastasis in patients with clinically N0 laryngeal cancer, rate of metastasis ranged between 0% and 3,2% (Koybasioglu, 2002, Aydogan, 2004, Coskun, 2004, Lim, 2006, Elsheikh, 2006, Paleri, 2008). In these studies, there was no isolated sublevel IIB metastasis and metastases in sublevel IIB were always associated with sublevel IIA metastases. Rinaldo et al (Rinaldo, 2006) reviewed the results of these studies and concluded that dissection of sublevel IIB is not indicated in patients with clinically N0 laryngeal cancer. The authors have concluded that spinal accessory nerve dysfunction can be minimized without reduction in the oncological safety of the neck dissection by this way. After oncological safety of level IIB preserving selective neck dissection for clinically N0 laryngeal cancer has been demonstrated, a prospective study to analyze the functional outcome of this approach was performed in the author of this chapter's department (Celik, 2009). According to the results of this study, none of the 30 patients who underwent sublevel IIB preserving selective neck dissections for clinically N0 laryngeal cancer developed shoulder syndrome in the post-operative period.

The necessity of dissection of level IV in patients with clinically N0 laryngeal cancer has been questioned recently. Dissection of level IV is not without complications, chylous fistula and phrenic nerve injury may occur. In a previous study by the author of this chapter revealed no metastasis in level IV of 113 neck dissection specimens collected from 71 patients with clinically N0 laryngeal cancer (Coskun, 2004). Elsheikh et al performed a prospective study and evaluated metastasis by pathological and molecular analysis is 31 patients with clinically N0 laryngeal cancer. The authors found only one metastasis in level IV (3,2%) in a patient with a T3N0 transglottic cancer (Elsheikh, 2006). The studies regarding metastases to level IV in patients with clinically N0 laryngeal cancer were later reviewed by Elsheikh et al (Elsheikh, 2006) and the authors have concluded that level IV metastases are rare in clinically N0 laryngeal cancer. But the authors have stressed that the larynx is divided into three compartments, which have different lymphatic drainage pathways and the extent of dissection should be individualized according to the location of the primary tumor. The final conclusion was that dissection of level IV might not be indicated in patients with glottic or supraglottic tumors but transglottic or subglottic tumors might well require level IV dissection.

Based on the observations from prospective studies regarding level IIB and level IV metastases in patients with clinically N0 laryngeal cancer, Ferlito et al (Ferlito, 2008) suggested level IIA-III dissection in patients with glottic and supraglottic cancers with clinically N0 neck. This approach appears to be the current treatment of choice.

Recently, Medina et al (Medina, 2011) performed a comprehensive review about central compartment dissection in laryngeal cancer. The authors have found evidence that level VI metastases were frequent in patients with primary subglottic carcinomas, advanced glottic and advanced supraglottic carcinomas and recommended elective treatment of level VI in these patients. In such patients, selective neck dissection should be extended to include level VI.

In summary, carcinomas arising from different compartments of the larynx have different patterns of lymph node metastasis. Current literature supports level IIA, III dissection is early supraglottic and glottic cancers. Level IV dissection is required in transglottic, primary subglottic cancers and glottic cancers with subglottic extension. Dissection should be extended to include level VI in patients with primary subglottic carcinomas, advanced glottic and advanced supraglottic carcinomas.

2.1.3 Selective neck dissection for oropharyngeal and hypopharyngeal cancer

Elective treatment of the neck in patients with oropharyngeal or hypopharyngeal cancer is not as clear as oral cavity or larynx. First of all, oropharyngeal and hypopharyngeal cancers are rare, as compared to oral cavity or laryngeal cancers and there is less data in the literature regarding the distribution of occult metastasis of these cancers. Second, in the past few decades, treatment of oropharyngeal and hypopharyngeal cancers has shifted from surgery to chemoradiation in many centers, reserving surgery for salvage. The reasons for this shift are the high sensitivity of these cancers to chemoradiation and the functional losses associated with surgery. Obviously there are patients who are not good candidates for chemoradiation or whose tumors can be managed with function preserving surgery but an important proportion of these patients receive non-surgical treatments. So, it is difficult to make conclusions about elective management of the clinically N0 neck in patients with oropharyngeal and hypopharyngeal cancer.

Oropharyngeal cancers usually drain into level II, III and IV lymph nodes, as well as retropharyngeal and parapharyngeal lymph nodes (Ferlito, 2006). In patients with clinically N0 oropharyngeal cancer level II-IV dissection would be appropriate. Paleri et al (Paleri, 2008) found metastases in level IIB of 5 patients in a group of 96 patients (5,2%) with clinically N0 oropharyngeal cancer. Similarly, Villaret et al (Villaret, 2007) reported that two metastases in level IIB in 32 neck dissection specimens (6%) of patients with oropharyngeal cancer. Lodder et al (Lodder, 2008) found only one metastasis (1%) in level IV in specimens of 92 selective neck dissections for oropharyngeal cancer. These findings reflect that a more limited dissection confined to levels IIA and III may be appropriate, as is the case in oral cavity cancers, but more prospective studies with higher number of patients are required.

Pyriform sinuses drain into the jugulodigastric lymph node and to the midjugular and spinal accessory chains. Inferior portion of the hypopharynx and postcricoid region drain into the paratracheal and paraesophageal nodes and to nodes in the supraclavicular fossa. Posterior hypopharyngeal wall drain into the retropharyngeal nodes and to the midjugular chain (Uppaluri & Sunwoo, 2010). In 1990 Candela et al (Candela, 1990) reported the analysis of neck dissection specimens of 333 patients with oropharyngeal or hypopharyngeal cancers. They found that levels II, III and IV were most frequently involved and isolated skip metastases out of these levels occurred only in one patient (0,3%). The authors have concluded that their data supports selective neck dissection in patients with clinically N0 neck. Weber et al (Weber, 1993) examined paratracheal dissection specimens of patients with larynx, hypopharynx and cervical esophagus cancers and found paratracheal metastases in three of 36 patients (8,2%) with hypopharyngeal primaries. In conclusion, paratracheal lymph node dissection along with levels II, III and IV appears to be the appropriate management in patients with clinically N0 hypopharyngeal cancer.

2.1.4 Selective neck dissection for squamous cell carcinoma of other head and neck primary sites

There is insufficient data regarding selective neck dissection for squamous cell carcinoma of other head and neck primary sites, such as paranasal sinuses, nasopharynx, skin, etc.

The routine management of recurrent or residual neck disease after radiotherapy (or chemo-radiation) in patients with nasopharyngeal carcinoma has been radical neck dissection for many years. Recently, Zhang et al (Zhang, 2011) reported their experience with recurrent or residual regional metastases of nasopharyngeal carcinoma. Patients with residual disease had a better outcome than the patients with recurrent disease. There were 70 patients with residual neck disease and 42 of these patients one single persistent lymph node during the course of the treatment. Though the researchers had performed radical neck dissection in every case, they have concluded that residual disease limited to one single lymph node might be managed with selective neck dissection.

Ebrahimi et al (Ebrahimi, 2010) analysed the distribution of lymph node metastases in 295 neck dissection specimens of 282 patients with cutaneous squamous cell carcinoma of the head and neck. According to the distribution of metastases, they concluded that selective neck dissection including level I–III for facial primaries, level II–III for anterior scalp and external ear primaries, and levels II–V for posterior scalp and neck primaries would be appropriate.

2.2 Selective neck dissection for malignant tumors of the head and neck other than squamous cell carcinoma

2.2.1 Selective neck dissection for malignant salivary gland tumors

Management of clinically N0 neck in patients with malignant salivary gland tumors is controversial. Because of the relative rarity of these tumors and the high variability in clinical behavior of different histopathological tumor types, which are very high in number, it is difficult to draw conclusions. Armstrong et al (Armstrong, 1992) found occult metastases in 34 of the 90 (38%) of the patients with clinically N0 salivary gland cancer who underwent elective neck dissection. Some authors (Armstrong 1992, Spiro 1986, Yu 1987) have found evidence that the risk of metastasis is related to the site of the primary tumor, with submandibular gland having the highest risk for metastasis followed by parotid and minor salivary gland tumors. Some histopathological types including undifferentiated carcinoma, squamous cell carcinoma, high-grade mucoepidermoid carcinoma, adenocarcinoma NOS, carcinoma ex pleomorphic adenoma, and salivary duct carcinoma are also associated with a higher incidence of occult metastasis (Armstrong 1992, Yu 1987, Bhattacharya 2002, Regis De Brito Santos 2001, Ferlito 2001). Armstrong et al (Armstrong, 1992) found that high-grade tumors had a high risk of occult metastases (49%) compared to low grade or intermediate tumors (7%). Recently, experience of a single institution from Japan about elective neck dissection in 77 patients with carcinoma of the parotid gland has been reported (Kawata, 2010). Lymph node metastases were found in 61,3% and 22,9% of the patients with high-grade and intermediate-grade tumors, respectively. There was no metastasis from low-grade tumors. 51 patients were initially staged as clinically N0 and 8 of these patients had occult metastases on histopathologic examination (15,7%). The authors had performed modified radical neck dissection for high-grade tumors and selective neck dissection (level I-III and VA) for other tumors, in this group of 51 patients with clinically negative neck, but the outcome after treatment was not reported. Of note, the accuracy of preoperative fine needle aspiration cytology of the parotid tumor was low (46,5% overall), especially in patients with intermediate or low-grade tumors (32,5%). Thus the authors recommended elective neck dissection in every patient with N0 malignant parotid tumor owing to the low accuracy of pre-operative diagnosis.

Based on these observations, it can be concluded that elective neck dissection is indicated in patients with high grade tumors, submandibular gland tumors and tumors of certain histopathologic type with clinically N0 neck. But owing to the low accuracy of preoperative fine needle aspiration cytology, elective neck dissection may well be indicated in every patient with clinically N0 malignant salivary gland tumor.

Extent of elective neck dissection is not clear in patients with clinically N0 salivary gland cancer. For parotid tumors, selective neck dissection of levels I-IV (or I-III plus VA, Kawata, 2010) and for submandibular and sublingual gland tumors dissection of levels I to III is recommended (Armstrong, 1992; Gold, 2005).

2.2.2 Selective neck dissection for thyroid cancer

Thyroid cancers are a heterogeneous group with different clinical behaviour but management of the neck is important for almost all types of thyroid cancer. The American Head and Neck Society and American Academy of Otolaryngology-Head and Neck Surgery have recommended Central (level VI) neck dissection with or without dissection of other levels for thyroid cancer (Robbins, 2002). However, there is still debate on the extent of the nodal dissection for optimal outcome.

Papillary thyroid carcinoma, which is one of the most common cancers of the human body, is the most common thyroid malignancy. Though the level VI lymph nodes are the first echelon nodes for papillary carcinoma, lateral metastases are also very common. Occult lateral metastasis rate was 55% in a study (Lim, 2011) and lateral metastases were associated with primary tumor size and the number of metastatic central lymph nodes. Recently, Patron et al. (Patron, 2011) reported a much lower rate of lateral metastases (18,6%) in a group of 131 patients with papillary thyroid carcinoma. In this series, metastasis rate was 2,9% in level IIB and 0% in level VA, thus the authors recommended dissection of levels IIA, III, IV and VB for papillary thyroid carcinoma with clinically negative neck. In contrast, Vayisoglu et al (Vayisoglu, 2010) found metastases in 22 of 47 neck dissections (46,8%) and incidence of the lateral metastases was much higher. Levels II, III, IV and V were involved in 12.7%, 25.5%, 38.2%, and 8.5% of the specimens respectively. Level IIB metastases were also very rare in this study (one of 47 neck dissections, 2,1%) and the authors have concluded that level IIB might be left undissected in selective neck dissections for papillary thyroid carcinoma.

Medullary carcinoma is an aggressive form of thyroid cancer. Rate of lymph node metastasis is much higher in medullary carcinoma. Oskam et al (Oskam, 2008) found lymph node metastases in 91% of the ipsilateral neck dissection specimens, 91% of the paratracheal dissections and 63% of the contralateral dissections. There were metastases in five of the twelve elective neck dissection specimens. High number of positive lymph nodes was associated with a poor prognosis. Dissection of levels II-V accompanied with central dissection is recommended in every patient with medullary carcinoma.

2.2.3 Selective neck dissection for head and neck melanoma

Malignant melanoma is another rare tumor of the head and neck region with a very poor prognosis. Clinically apparent metastases of melanoma are treated with comprehensive neck dissection, however there is no consensus on how to treat the occult metastases. There are reports about sentinel node studies but the extent of dissection is not clear. Current literature supports comprehensive neck dissections rather than selective dissections, in order to achieve better regional control and adjuvant radiotherapy for patients with two or more involved lymph nodes (Hamming-Vrieze, 2009).

2.3 Selective neck dissection for clinically positive neck

The widely accepted management of clinically positive neck has been radical or modified neck dissection for several decades. Recently, some investigators have found strong evidence that selective neck dissection may be used for carefully selected patients with clinically positive necks. Andersen et al (Andersen, 2002) reported the results of 129 selective neck dissections in 106 patients with previously untreated head and neck cancer and clinically positive neck. They obtained a regional control rate of 94,3% with six recurrences in the operated side of the neck that had undergone selective neck dissection. Kowalski and Carvalho (Kowalski & Carvalho, 2002) retrospectively analyzed radical neck dissection specimens of 164 patients with oral cavity cancer and clinically N1 or N2a neck. They found only one metastasis in level IV (0,6%) and none at level V. They also noted a high false positive rate (57,4% pN0) in N1 patients with the clinically positive node in level I. The authors have concluded that supraomohyoid neck dissection may be used instead of radical neck dissection in patients with clinically N1 neck in level I. More recently Santos et al (Santos, 2006) reported their results of 34 selective neck dissections performed on 28 patients with clinically N+ head and neck cancer. They had four recurrences (11,8%) after selective neck dissection. One of these patients was N1, two were N2b and one was N2c. Three of these patients had T4 tumors and one had T3 tumor. Researchers from University of Pittsburgh (Simental, 2006) performed a retrospective analysis of 65 patients with clinically N+ head and neck cancer who underwent selective neck dissection. There were 8 recurrences (12,3%), four of them occurred outside the field of dissection and four recurrences (6,1%) occurred in the field of dissection. Four recurrences could be managed by salvage surgery with a resultant overall regional control rate of 93,9%. In this series, 21 of the 65 cases (%32) who were staged clinically N+ did not have metastasis on pathological examination.

In a recent study (Dhiwakar, 2010), it has been reported that selective neck dissection can be used to treat clinically positive neck with involvement of non-lymphatic structures, especially if the nodal disease was confined to two or less neck levels. The authors were able to obtain a recurrence rate of 0% for primary treatment cases and 13% for post-radiation cases. Though these results are very encouraging, this is the only study reported in this specific group of disease and needs to be supported with further studies.

It should be noted the two of the studies mentioned above (Santos, 2006; Simental, 2006) reported relatively high rates of regional failure and reflect undertreatment in these patients. Obviously an important proportion of patients with clinically N+ neck do not have metastasis on histopathological examination and any neck treatment would be an overtreatment for these patients, but a balance between overtreatment and undertreatment should be implemented. Based on the observations from the current literature, it appears that selective neck dissection is feasible in some carefully selected patients with clinically positive neck. However, more prospective and primary site-specific studies with larger number of patients are needed to identify which patients with clinically N+ neck are good candidates for selective neck dissections.

2.4 Selective neck dissection after primary chemo-radiation for head and neck cancer

Planned radical neck dissection for initially positive neck after completion of primary chemo-radiation, regardless of the initial stage and response of the neck disease was the treatment of choice in the first years of the age of organ preservation. In the following years, there has been a consensus that planned neck dissection in patients who initially present with N1 neck disease is not necessary. However, debate continues about routine performance of planned neck dissection for patients who present initially with bulky (≥N2) neck disease. Recently Ferlito et al (Ferlito, 2010) reviewed the literature to evaluate the necessity of planned neck dissection after complete response to chemo-radiation. The authors have found 24 articles in favour of benefit of planned neck dissection and 26 articles that do not demonstrate an advantage of planned neck dissection. The authors have concluded that use of planned neck dissection for patients with a complete response to chemo-radiation cannot be justified.

Nowadays, it has been demonstrated that selective neck dissection is possible in some of these patients. Langerman et al (Langerman, 2009) performed 43 neck dissections on 34 patients after completion chemo-radiotherapy. All patients had N2 or greater disease before treatment and 39 of the 43 neck dissections (91%) performed were selective neck dissections. In this study post-treatment computed tomography was used to determine the extent of neck dissection and was found to be helpful. More recently, Dhiwakar (Dhiwakar, 2011) reported their results of selective neck dissection performed for persistent neck disease following chemoradiation. Sixty-nine selective neck dissections were performed on 62 patients and only one recurrence was observed. Another study supporting selective neck dissection after chemo-radiation was presented by Cannady et al (Cannady, 2010). The authors have demonstrated that SND would remove residual disease in most cases when the dissection would encompass the next distal level with the original levels.

In summary, the current literature does not support planned neck dissection after complete response to chemo-radiation. In the case of persistent neck disease, selective neck dissection is feasible in the majority of the cases.

2.5 Surgical technique of selective neck dissection

The first step of selective neck dissection is the skin incision. In most instances, neck dissection is performed along with a primary tumor removal and an incision, which allows primary tumor removal and neck dissection is preferred. If the plan is to perform a laryngectomy with bilateral neck dissections a "U" shaped incision is used to create an apron flap. In other instances, the author of this chapter prefers a "MacFee incision". In most instances a single horizontal incision placed at the level of thyroid notch or cricoid cartilage allows removal of all lymph node groups, but occasionally two incisions, one at the level of the hyoid bone and one 2-3 cm above the clavicle, may be necessary. Especially if removal the primary tumor requires a lip split incision, two horizontal incisions are used and the upper incision is combined with the lip split incision. For a unilateral neck dissection the incision extends from a point 3-4 cm posterior to the sternocleidomastoid (SCM) muscle to a point on the 3-4 cm other side of the midline. For bilateral neck dissection, the incision extends 3-4 cm posterior to the SCM on each side. The superior and inferior skin flaps are elevated in a subplatysmal plane to allow exposure of the border of the mandible superiorly and the clavicle inferiorly. If level IV will not be dissected, elevation of the inferior flap down to the level of cricoid cartilage is sufficient. After the skin flaps are elevated, the superficial layer of the deep cervical fascia overlying the submandibular gland is incised at the inferior border of the gland and elevated as a second layer up to the level of the border of the mandible in order to protect the marginal mandibular branch of the facial nerve, which lies within this fascia.

Next, the investing layer of the deep cervical fascia is incised along the anterior border of the SCM. Fascia on the lateral surface of the SCM must be protected, not peeled off. This fascia prevents scar formation and adhesion of the SCM to platysma and overlying skin. Preservation of the fascia may help to reduce post-operative shoulder pain. The external jugular vein may need to be divided and ligated at the level of angle of the mandible but it is better protected whenever possible. The SCM is retracted laterally and posteriorly while the fibro-fatty tissue of the anterior triangle of the neck is retracted medially, allowing an easy dissection during clearance of levels II, III and if necessary level IV along the anterior and medial surface of the SCM. As the fibro-fatty tissue is peeled off the SCM, the spinal accessory nerve (SAN) comes into view in the junction of upper and middle thirds of the SCM. For easier dissection at level II, the investing layer of the deep cervical fascia is divided at the inferior border of the posterior belly of the digastric muscle and the muscle is retracted medially and superiorly for a good exposure. Then the fibro-fatty tissue overlying the spinal accessory nerve is dissected off the nerve up to the skull base. This is done by opening up the tissues with a fine tipped haemostat and cutting the tissues with a scalpel. After the nerve is traced up to the skull base, all the fibro-fatty tissue should be cut with a scalpel down to the fascia of deep neck muscles along the course of the nerve. Very rarely, internal carotid artery may be tortuous at this level mimicking a lymph node and causing a big danger. The fibro-fatty tissue posterior to the SAN is level IIB and after freeing from the surrounding structures, this tissue is passed under the SAN and brought into level IIA. However, this manoeuvre requires traction of the SAN, which may result in dysfunction of the nerve. It is better to remove level IIB separately and continue with dissection of level IIA without traction of the SAN. Dissection is continued along the posterior border of SCM to the inferior extent of dissection, either to clavicle or the tendon of the omohyoid muscle. Traction of the SCM should be minimized. Pulling the fibro-fatty tissue medially with haemostats placed in multiple points and retracting the SCM laterally with gauze hold by the primary surgeon's left hand can achieve a good exposure. During this dissection, branches of the cervical plexus are encountered and protected. The first three roots give fibers to the spinal accessory nerve and cutting these roots cause dysfunction of the nerve. Also preservation of the cervical roots prevents numbness of the neck skin and may help to reduce shoulder pain.

After the dissection along the posterior border of the SCM is completed, the fibro-fatty is grasped from several points with haemostats and pulled in a lateral and anterior direction by an assistant. In an "en bloc" fashion, all the fibro-fatty tissue is dissected over the branches of the cervical plexus in an anterior direction using a scalpel. Sharp dissection continues over the carotid sheath but care is taken not to injure the carotid artery, the vagus nerve and the internal jugular vein. The internal jugular vein is very fragile and must never be hold with an instrument with sharp teeth. The vein has many branches along its course and all these branches need to be clamped and suture ligated. Also every effort should be made to visualize and protect the lymphatic duct in level IV, which is constantly present on the left side and frequently present on the right side of the neck. The fibro-fatty tissue lying medial to the carotid sheath is dissected to the lateral border of the strap muscles, which is the medial border of dissection. Care must be taken to protect the superior laryngeal nerve at this point.

If level I is to be dissected, dissection continues upward. The medial border of the anterior belly of the opposite digastric muscle and the inferior border of the mandible are the borders of level I dissection. The fibro-fatty tissue is grasped with haemostats in several points and cleared over the underlying muscles. In most instances the submandibular gland is removed along with the fibro-fatty tissue. Although the gland is almost never involved with disease and there are authors who recommend preservation of the gland, to assure a complete removal of all submandibular lymph nodes excision of the gland is usually required. All the fibro-fatty tissue down to the mylohyoid muscle must be cleared.

During the whole dissection, use of mono-polar cautery should be minimized in order to avoid heat damage to the nerves in the surgical field. Bi-polar cautery should be used whenever haemostasis is necessary.

After completion of dissection two vacuum drains, one anterior to the carotid sheath and one posterior to the sheath are placed and secured. Subcutaneous layer and skin is closed in the usual fashion.

3. Conclusion

Presence of cervical lymph node metastases is one of the most important prognostic factors of head and neck cancer. Since the first introduction for more than 100 years ago, neck dissection has been the main treatment of clinically apparent or occult lymph node metastases. Through decades, the procedure of neck dissection has undergone an evolution. Today, neck dissection limited to only the lymph node levels, which contain or at high risk for metastases, can offer very good regional control rates. Recent studies have clearly demonstrated that level IIB and V can be left undissected in the majority of head and neck cancers. There is also evidence that level IV dissection can be omitted in some patients. These modifications help to avoid complications such as spinal accessory nerve dysfunction or chylous fistula. On the other hand, for some patients, lymph node levels which are not routinely dissected during neck dissection, such as level VI or retropharyngeal lymph nodes need to be addressed to achieve regional control. Head and neck cancer is not a homogenous disease and neck dissection has to be individualized every patient. This requires a thorough knowledge of embryology, anatomy and pattern of lymphatic drainage for every anatomic subsite and clinical behaviour of cancer originating in these subsites.
The very recent classification of neck dissection proposed by Ferlito and colleagues offers a big flexibility and apparently will soon gain worldwide acceptance.

4. Acknowledgment

I would like to thank to my teachers in Uludag University School of Medicine Department of Otolaryngology, Professors Metin Arat, Ilker Tezel, Ibrahim Hizalan, Selcuk Onart and Levent Erisen, for teaching and supporting me since the time I started my residency training in the department.

5. References

Andersen PE, Warren F, Spiro J, Burningham A, Wong R, Wax MK, Shah JP, Cohen JI. Results of selective neck dissection in management of the node-positive neck. Arch Otolaryngol Head Neck Surg. 2002 Oct;128(10):1180-4.

Armstrong JG, Harrison LB, Thaler HT, et al: The indications for elective treatment of the neck in cancer of the major salivary glands. Cancer 1992; 69:615-619.

Armstrong WB, Netterville JL: Anatomy of the larynx, trachea, and bronchi. *Otolaryngol Clin North Am* 1995; 28:685-699.

Ayad T, Guertin L, Soulières D, Belair M, Temam S, Nguyen-Tân PF. Controversies in the management of retromolar trigone carcinoma. Head Neck. 2009 Mar;31(3):398-405.

Aydogan LB, Aydogan FK, Uguz A, et al. Levels IIB and IV in- volvement in laryngeal carcinoma. Final Program and Abstract Book, 6th International Conference on Head Neck Cancer, Washington, DC, 2004: 111 (poster session 1, p 1–195)

Bajwa MS, McMillan R, Khattak O, Thomas M, Krishnan OP, Webster K. Neck recurrence after level I-IV or I-III selective neck dissection in the management of the clinically N0 neck in patients with oral squamous cell carcinoma. Head Neck. 2011 Mar;33(3):403-6.

Bhattacharyya N, Fried MP: Nodal metastasis in major salivary gland cancer: predictive factors and effects on survival. Arch Otolaryngol Head Neck Surg 2002; 128:904-908.

Brazilian Head and Neck Cancer Study Group. Results of a prospective trial on elective modified radical classical versus supraomohyoid neck dissection in the management of oral squamous carcinoma. Am J Surg. 1998 Nov;176(5):422-7.

Byers RM, Weber RS, Andrews T, McGill D, Kare R, Wolf P. Frequency and therapeutic implications of "skip metastases" in the neck from squamous carcinoma of the oral tongue. Head Neck 1997;19:14–9.

Byers RM. (1985). Modified neck dissection. A study of 967 cases from 1970 to 1980. *Am J Surg,* Vol. 150, No. 4, (October 1985), pp. (414–421), ISSN 0002-9610

Candela FC, Kothari K, Shah JP. Patterns of cervical node metastases from squamous carcinoma of the oropharynx and hypopharynx. Head Neck. 1990 May-Jun;12(3):197-203.

Cannady SB, Lee WT, Scharpf J, Lorenz RR, Wood BG, Strome M, Lavertu P, Esclamado RM, Saxton JP, Adelstein DJ. Extent of neck dissection required after concurrent chemoradiation for stage IV head and neck squamous cell carcinoma. Head Neck. 2010 Mar;32(3):348-56.

Celik B, Coskun H, Kumas FF, Irdesel J, Zarifoglu M, Erisen L, Onart S. Accessory nerve function after level 2b-preserving selective neck dissection. Head Neck. 2009 Nov;31(11):1496-501.

Coskun HH, Erisen L, Basut O. Selective neck dissection for clinically N0 neck in laryngeal cancer: is dissection of level IIb necessary? Otolaryngol Head Neck Surg 2004;131:655–659.

De Zinis LO, Bolzoni A, Piazza C, Nicolai P. Prevalence and localization of nodal metastases in squamous cell carcinoma of the oral cavity: role and extension of neck dissection. Eur Arch Otorhinolaryngol. 2006 Dec;263(12):1131-5.

Dhiwakar M, Robbins KT, Rao K, Vieira F, Malone J. Efficacy of selective neck dissection for nodal metastasis with involvement of nonlymphatic structures.Head Neck. 2011 Aug;33(8):1099-105

Dhiwakar M, Robbins KT, Vieira F, Rao K, Malone J. Selective neck dissection as an early salvage intervention for clinically persistent nodal disease following chemoradiation. Head Neck. 2011 Apr 5. doi: 10.1002/hed.21707. [Epub ahead of print]

Dias FL, Lima RA, Kligerman J, Farias TP, Soares JR, Manfro G, Sa GM. Relevance of skip metastases for squamous cell carcinoma of the oral tongue and the floor of the mouth. Otolaryngol Head Neck Surg. 2006 Mar;134(3):460-5.

Ebrahimi A, Moncrieff MD, Clark JR, Shannon KF, Gao K, Milross CG, O'Brien CJ. Predicting the pattern of regional metastases from cutaneous squamous cell carcinoma of the head and neck based on location of the primary. Head Neck. 2010 Oct;32(10):1288-94.

Elsheikh MN, Mahfouz ME, Elsheikh E. Level IIb lymph nodes metastasis in elective supraomohyoid neck dissection for oral cavity squamous cell carcinoma: a molecular-based study. Laryngoscope. 2005 Sep;115(9):1636-40.

Elsheikh MN, Ferlito A, Rinaldo A, Shaha AR, Khafif A, Coskun HH, Kowalski LP, Medina JE. Do pathologic and molecular analyses of neck dissection specimens justify the preservation of level IV for laryngeal squamous carcinoma with clinically negative neck? J Am Coll Surg. 2006 Feb;202(2):320-3.

Elsheikh MN, Mahfouz ME, Salim EI, Elsheikh EA. Molecular assessment of neck dissections supports preserving level IIB lymph nodes in selective neck dissection for laryngeal squamous cell carcinoma with a clinically negative neck. ORL J Otorhinolaryngol Relat Spec 2006;68:177–184.

Erisen L, Basel B, Coskun H, et al. Evaluation of the number of lymph nodes dissected and neck recurrences in comprehensive and selective neck dissections. Kulak Burun Bogaz Ihtis Derg 2001;8:391-6 [Turkish].

Erisen L, Basel B, Irdesel J, et al. Shoulder function after accessory nerve-sparing neck dissections. Head Neck. 2004 Nov;26(11):967-71.

Fakih AR, Rao RS, Borges AM, Patel AR. Elective versus therapeutic neck dissection in early carcinoma of the oral tongue. Am J Surg 1989;158:309 – 313

Fasunla AJ, Greene BH, Timmesfeld N, Wiegand S, Werner JA, Sesterhenn AM. A meta-analysis of the randomized controlled trials on elective neck dissection versus therapeutic neck dissection in oral cavity cancers with clinically node-negative neck. Oral Oncol. 2011 May;47(5):320-4.

Ferlito A, Buckley JG, Shaha AR, et al. Rationale for selective neck dissection in tumors of upper aerodigestive tract. Acta Otolaryngol 2001;121:548-55.

Ferlito A, Shaha AR, Rinaldo A, et al: Management of clinically negative cervical lymph nodes in patients with malignant neoplasms of the parotid gland. ORL; J Otorhinolaryngol Rel Spec 2001; 63:123-126.

Ferlito, A & Rinaldo, A. (2004). Osvaldo Suarez : Often-Forgotten father of Functional Neck Dissection (in the Non-Spanish-Speaking Literature. *Laryngoscope,* Vol. 114, No. 7, (July 2004), pp. (1177-1178), ISSN 1531-4995

Ferlito A, Rinaldo A, Silver CE, et al: Effective and therapeutic selective neck dissection. Oral Oncol 2006; 42:14-25.

Ferlito A, Silver CE, Rinaldo A. Selective neck dissection (IIA, III): a rational replacement for complete functional neck dissection in patients with N0 supraglottic and glottic squamous carcinoma. Laryngoscope. 2008 Apr;118(4):676-9.

Ferlito A, Corry J, Silver CE, Shaha AR, Thomas Robbins K, Rinaldo A. Planned neck dissection for patients with complete response to chemoradiotherapy: a concept approaching obsolescence. Head Neck. 2010 Feb;32(2):253-61.

Ferlito A, Robbins KT, Shah JP, Medina JE, Silver CE, Al-Tamimi S, Fagan JJ, et al. Proposal for a rational classification of neck dissections. Head Neck. 2011 Mar;33(3):445-50

Godden DR, Ribeiro NF, Hassanein K, Langton SG. Recurrent neck disease in oral cancer. J Oral MaxillofacSurg 2002;60:748 – 753.

Gold DR, Annino Jr DJ: Management of the neck in salivary gland carcinoma. Otolaryngol Clin North Am 2005; 38:99-105.

Hamming-Vrieze O, Balm AJ, Heemsbergen WD, Hooft van Huysduynen T, Rasch CR. Regional control of melanoma neck node metastasis after selective neck dissection with or without adjuvant radiotherapy. Arch Otolaryngol Head Neck Surg. 2009 Aug;135(8):795-800.

Jones AS, Roland NJ, Field JK, et al. The level of cervical lymph node metastases: their prognostic relevance and relationship with head and neck squamous carcinoma primary sites. Clin Otolar- yngol 1994;19:63-9.

Jones KR, Lodge-Rigal RD, Reddick RL, Tudor GE, Shockley WW. Prognostic factors in the recurrence of stage I and II squamous cell cancer of the oral cavity. Arch Otolaryngol Head Neck Surg 1992;118:483 – 485.

Kawata R, Koutetsu L, Yoshimura K, Nishikawa S, Takenaka H. Indication for elective neck dissection for N0 carcinoma of the parotid gland: a single institution's 20-year experience. Acta Otolaryngol. 2010 Feb;130(2):286-92.

Kligerman J, Lima RA, Soares JR, et al. Supraomohyoid neck dissection in the treatment of T1/T2 squamous cell carcinoma of oral cavity. Am J Surg 1994;168:391 - 394.

Kowalski LP, Franco EL, de Andrade Sobrinho J. Factors influencing regional lymph node metastasis from laryngeal carcinoma. Ann Otol Rhinol Laryngol 1995;104:442-7.

Kowalski LP, Carvalho AL. Feasibility of supraomohyoid neck dissection in N1 and N2a oral cancer patients. Head Neck. 2002 Oct;24(10):921-4.

Koybasioglu A, Tokcaer AB, Uslu S, et al. Accessory nerve function after modified radical and lateral neck dissections. Laryngoscope 2000;110:73-7.

Koybasioglu A, Uslu S, Yilmaz M, et al. Lymphatic metastasis to the supraretrospinal recess in laryngeal squamous cell carcinoma. Ann Otol Rhinol Laryngol 2002;111:96–99.

Lea J, Bachar G, Sawka AM, Lakra DC, Gilbert RW, Irish JC, Brown DH, Gullane PJ, Goldstein DP. Metastases to level IIb in squamous cell carcinoma of the oral cavity: a systematic review and meta-analysis. Head Neck. 2010 Feb;32(2):184-90.

Lim YC, Lee JS, Koo BS, Choi EC. Level IIb lymph node metastasis in laryngeal squamous cell carcinoma. Laryngoscope 2006;116:268–272.

Lim YS, Lee JC, Lee YS, Lee BJ, Wang SG, Son SM, Kim IJ. Lateral cervical lymph node metastases from papillary thyroid carcinoma: predictive factors of nodal metastasis. Surgery. 2011 Jul;150(1):116-21.

Lodder WL, Sewnaik A, den Bakker MA, Meeuwis CA, Kerrebijn JD. Selective neck dissection for N0 and N1 oral cavity and oropharyngeal cancer: are skip metastases a real danger? Clin Otolaryngol. 2008 Oct;33(5):450-7.

Medina JE, Ferlito A, Robbins KT, Silver CE, Rodrigo JP, de Bree R, Rinaldo A, Elsheikh MN, Weber RS, Werner JA. Central compartment dissection in laryngeal cancer. Head Neck. 2011 May;33(5):746-52.

Mishra P, Sharma AK. A 3-year study of supraomohyoid neck dissection and modified radical neck dissection type I in oral cancer: with special reference to involvement of level IV node metastasis. Eur Arch Otorhinolaryngol. 2010 Jun;267(6):933-8.

Oskam IM, Hoebers F, Balm AJ, van Coevorden F, Bais EM, Hart AM, van den Brekel MW. Neck management in medullary thyroid carcinoma. Eur J Surg Oncol. 2008 Jan;34(1):71-6.

Paleri V, Kumar Subramaniam S, Oozeer N, Rees G, Krishnan S. Dissection of the submuscular recess (sublevel IIb) in squamous cell cancer of the upper aerodigestive tract: prospective study and systematic review of the literature. Head Neck. 2008 Feb;30(2):194-200.

Pentenero M, Gandolfo S, Carrozzo M. Importance of tumor thickness and depth of invasion in nodal involvement and prognosis of oral squamous cell carcinoma: a review of the literature. Head Neck. 2005 Dec;27(12):1080-91.

Po Wing Yuen A, Lam KY, Lam LK, Ho CM, Wong A, Chow TL, Yuen WF, Wei WI. Prognostic factors of clinically stage I and II oral tongue carcinoma-A comparative study of stage, thickness, shape, growth pattern, invasive front malignancy grading, Martinez-Gimeno score, and pathologic features. Head Neck. 2002 Jun;24(6):513-20.

Razfar A, Walvekar RR, Melkane A, Johnson JT, Myers EN. Incidence and patterns of regional metastasis in early oral squamous cell cancers: feasibility of submandibular gland preservation. Head Neck. 2009 Dec;31(12):1619-23.

Regis De Brito Santos I, Kowalski LP, Cavalcante De Araujo V, etal: Multivariate analysis of risk factors for neck metastases in surgically treated parotid carcinomas. Arch Otolaryngol Head Neck Surg 2001; 127:56-60. 179.

Rinaldo A, Elsheikh MN, Ferlito A, et al. Prospective studies of neck dissection specimens support preservation of sublevel IIB for laryngeal squamous carcinoma with clinically negative neck. J Am Coll Surg. 2006 Jun;202(6):967-70.

Robbins KT, Medina JE, Wolfe GT, Levine PA, Sessions RB, Pruet CW: Standardizing neck dissection terminology. Official report of the Academy's Committee for Head and Neck Sur- gery and Oncology. *Arch Otolaryngol Head Neck Surg* 1991, 117:601-605.

Robbins KT, Clayman G, Levine PA, et al. American Head and Neck Society. American Academy of Otolaryngology–Head and Neck Surgery. Neck dissection classification update: revisions proposed by the American Head and Neck Society and the American Academy of Otolaryngology–Head and Neck Surgery. Arch Otolaryngol Head Neck Surg 2002;128:751-8.

Ross GL, Soutar DS, MacDonald DG, Shoaib T, Camilleri IG, Robertson AG. Improved staging of cervical metastases in clinically node-negative patients with head and neck squamous cell carcinoma. Ann Surg Oncol 2004;11: 213 – 218.

Santos AB, Cernea CR, Inoue M, Ferraz AR. Selective neck dissection for node-positive necks in patients with head and neck squamous cell carcinoma: a word of caution. Arch Otolaryngol Head Neck Surg. 2006 Jan;132(1):79-81.

Sheahan P, O'Keane C, Sheahan JN, O'Dwyer TP. Effect of tumor thickness and other factors on the risk of regional disease and treatment of the N0 neck in early oral squamous carcinoma. Clin Otolaryngol 2003;28: 461 – 471.

Sparano A, Weinstein G, Chalian A, Yodul M, Weber R. Multivariate predictors of occult neck metastasis in early oral tongue cancer. Otolaryngol Head Neck Surg 2004; 131:472 – 476.

Spiro RH, Huvos AG, Wong GY, Spiro JD, Gnecco CA, Strong EW. Predictive value of tumor thickness in squamous carcinoma confined to the tongue and floor of the mouth. Am J Surg 1986;152:345 – 350.

Spiro RH: Salivary neoplasms: overview of a 35-year experience with 2,807 patients. Head Neck Surg 1986; 8:177-184.

Uppaluri, R & Sunwoo, JB. (2010). Neoplasms of the Hypopharynx and Cervical Esophagus, In : *Cummings Otolaryngology Head & Neck Surgery,* Flint PW, Haughey BH, Lund VJ, Niparko JK, Richardson MA, Thomas JR, pp. 1177-1230, Mosby Elsevier, ISBN 978-0-323-05283-2, Philadelphia.

Villaret AB, Piazza C, Peretti G, Calabrese L, Ansarin M, Chiesa F, Pellini R, Spriano G, Nicolai P. Multicentric prospective study on the prevalence of sublevel IIb metastases in head and neck cancer. Arch Otolaryngol Head Neck Surg. 2007 Sep;133(9):897-903.

Weber RS, Marvel J, Smith P, et al: Paratracheal lymph node dissection for carcinoma of the larynx, hypopharynx, and cervical esophagus. Otolaryngol Head Neck Surg 1993; 108:11.

Woolgar JA. T2 carcinoma of the tongue: the histopathologist's perspective. Br J Oral Maxillofac Surg 1999;37: 187 – 193.

Woolgar JA. Salvage neck dissections in oral and oropharyngeal squamous cell carcinoma: histological features in relation to disease category. Int J Oral Maxillofac Surg. 2006 Oct;35(10):907-12.

Yu GY, Ma DQ: Carcinoma of the salivary gland: a clinicopathologic study of 405 cases. Semin Surg Oncol 1987; 3:240-244.

Zhang L, Zhu YX, Wang Y, Huang CP, Wu Y, Ji QH. Salvage surgery for neck residue or recurrence of nasopharyngeal carcinoma: a 10-year experience. Ann Surg Oncol. 2011 Jan;18(1):233-8